For Butterworth-Heinemann:

Commissioning Editor: Susan Young
Development Editor: Catherine Jackson
Project Manager: Gail Wright
Designer: George Ajayi

Regulating Healthcare Quality: Legal and Professional Issues

Edited by

John Tingle BA Law(Hons) CertEd MEd Barrister

Reader in Health Law, Director of the Centre for Health Law, Nottingham Law School,
The Nottingham Trent University, Nottingham, UK

Charles Foster MA(Cantab) VetMB MRCVS, of the Inner Temple,
Barrister

Barrister at 6 Pump Court, Temple, London, UK

Kay Wheat BA Solicitor

Reader in Law, Nottingham Law School, The Nottingham Trent University, Nottingham, UK

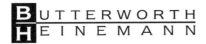

EDINBURGH LONDON NEW YORK OXFORD PHILADELPHIA ST LOUIS SYDNEY TORONTO 2004

BUTTERWORTH-HEINEMANN
An imprint of Elsevier Limited

First published 2004

ISBN 0 7506 8784 3

British Library Cataloguing in Publication Data
A catalogue record for this book is available from the British Library

Library of Congress Cataloging in Publication Data
A catalog record for this book is available from the Library of Congress

Notice
Medical knowledge is constantly changing. Standard safety precautions must be followed, but as new research and clinical experience broaden our knowledge, changes in treatment and drug therapy may become necessary or appropriate. Readers are advised to check the most current product information provided by the manufacturer of each drug to be administered to verify the recommended dose, the method and duration of administration, and contraindications. It is the responsibility of the practitioner, relying on experience and knowledge of the patient, to determine dosages and the best treatment for each individual patient. Neither the Publisher nor the editors assume any liability for any injury and/or damage to persons or property arising from this publication.

The Publisher

 your source for books,
journals and multimedia
in the health sciences

www.elsevierhealth.com

The
Publisher's
policy is to use
**paper manufactured
from sustainable forests**

Printed in China

Contents

List of Contributors

Troyen A. Brennan MD JD MPH
Professor of Law and Public Health, Department of Health Policy and Management, Harvard School of Public Health; Professor of Medicine, Department of Medicine, Harvard Medical School; Department of Medicine, Brigham & Women's Hospital, Boston, USA

Richard Burchill BA (Maine) BA (Hull) PhD (Nottingham)
Lecturer, Law School; Director, McCaubrey Centre for International Law, University of Hull, Hull, UK

Helen Caulfield LLB(Hons) MA(Hons) MSc(Hons)
Policy Advisor, Royal College of Nursing, London, UK

Charles Foster MA(Cantab) VetMB MRCVS, of the Inner Temple, Barrister
Barrister at 6 Pump Court, Temple, London, UK

Keith Haynes LLB(Hons) MSc DipHSM
Director of MPS Risk Consulting, Leeds; Visiting Senior Lecturer, Department of Health Sciences, University of York, York; Honorary Fellow, Faculty of Medicine, University of Manchester, Manchester, UK

Stephen Heasell BA(Hons) CNAA
Head of Division of Economics, Faculty of Economics and Social Sciences, The Nottingham Trent University, Nottingham, UK

Timothy James BA CertEd
Senior Lecturer, Law School, University of Central England, Birmingham, UK

Carolyn Johnston LLB LLM MA
Project Officer to the UK Clinical Ethics Network (Ethox), University of Oxford, Oxford; Senior Lecturer, School of Law, Kingston University, Kingston-upon-Thames, UK

Susan Kerrison MSc
Honorary Senior Research Fellow, Public Health Policy Research Unit, School of Public Policy, UCL, London; Assistant Director (Research Governance), University College London NHS Trust, London, UK

Michelle M. Mello JD PhD MPhil
Assistant Professor of Health Policy and Law, Department of Health Policy and Management, Harvard School of Public Health, Boston, USA

Duncan Pratt BA(Oxon) Barrister
Barrister at Chambers of Kieran Coonan QC, 6 Pump Court, Temple, London, UK

John Tingle BA Law(Hons) CertEd MEd Barrister
Reader in Health Law, Director of the Centre for Health Law, Nottingham Law School, The Nottingham Trent University, Nottingham, UK

Kay Wheat BA Solicitor
Reader in Law, Nottingham Law School, The Nottingham Trent University, Nottingham, UK

Elizabeth Wicks LLB LLM PhD
Lecturer in Law, University of Birmingham, Birmingham, UK

Preface

This book is concerned with the interface between health regulation, healthcare quality, law and ethics. The subject area is vast and diverse, and rapidly developing. In order to provide a detailed coverage of issues, we invited contributors from a wide range of health-related disciplines. The book chapters fully reflect the interrelated nature of health regulation and health quality.

The government has stated that improvement of the quality of healthcare provision in the NHS is an urgent priority, and certainly a lot of money and effort is devoted to it. It is repeatedly asserted that the NHS exists for the patient, not the patient for the NHS. Concepts like 'patient empowerment' increasingly dominate policy: whether they dominate practice is another matter. Many organisations now purport to regulate and ensure healthcare quality. Anyone working in health care has to be able to navigate through a dense jungle of acronyms: NICE, CHI, CHAI, NPSA, NHSLA, CNST, PALS, CPPIH and OSCS are just a few examples.

All these organisations have to operate within the context of an adversarial, tort-based, civil compensation system. Patients today expect far more from their carers than they used to. They are less deferential and less forgiving: they are very ready to limp straight out of hospital to their solicitor. All these factors have created a tense, angst-ridden but legally and ethically fascinating healthcare environment. It is that environment which we explore in this book.

John Tingle
Charles Foster
Kay Wheat

Nottingham and London, 2004

Table of Cases

United Kingdom Cases

European Commission and Court of Human Rights

Other Jurisdictions

Canada

New Zealand

United States

Table of Statutes

Table of Statutory Instruments

Table of Conventions and International Instruments

Introduction

John Tingle

REGULATION AS A CONCEPT

Regulation as a concept has been interpreted broadly within this book with macro and micro perspectives being adopted. A number of chapters concentrate on the legal regulation of specific issues such as clinical negligence litigation (hard regulation), while others focus on regulation through government initiatives such as clinical governance and the NHS complaints system (soft regulation). All the chapters in this book reveal the complexity of the issues involved with regulating the NHS and in particular healthcare quality. The system of quality regulation appears almost organic and very finely balanced.

Regulation of health and healthcare quality can be seen to be carried out by the courts when they decide cases and award compensation to patients injured by negligent practice. Regulation of health and health quality also takes place within the NHS. Clinical governance, controls assurance and clinical risk management are just some of the government NHS policy initiatives in this area.

In the courts, the sanction for breach is monetary compensation called damages. Outside the courts, the health inspectorate, CHI (Commission for Health Improvement) makes sure that the government health quality initiatives are being taken seriously by NHS trusts and the sanction for breach can be adverse publicity and shame caused by the publication of damning and critical CHI reports.

All these pressures combine to secure the accountability of the NHS to the public and to regulate health care and to ensure health quality.

A complex NHS

In reading the chapters in this book, it should not be forgotten that the NHS is a vast and complex place, comprising many sets of organisations with different types of staff, all maintaining differing agendas and work cultures. It would seem from the discussions in some of the chapters that ingrained NHS work cultures cannot be changed overnight. A well-regulated, safe and quality-based healthcare culture must be nurtured and developed incrementally. Effective regulation of the NHS can be seen to be taking place and the quality of health care is improving, but perhaps the pace of change is not fast enough. A review of CHI inspection reports confirms this view. CHI in its latest annual report[1] states:

'CHI's reports show that while organisations are working better together and there are some good examples of organisations running their services more effectively, too often care is still organised around the convenience of the NHS rather than the people who use the service.'

CHI looked at emerging themes from 175 clinical governance reviews[2] and stated:

'Risk Management: Many trusts are poor at managing potential risks to patients and many staff fear reprisals if they reported things going wrong. The risks can be made worse by staff shortages and poor attendance on mandatory training courses.'

'Soft' regulation, such as clinical governance and clinical risk management can be viewed to be working as a regulator of NHS health care; the difficulty is to definitively prove the extent of this with scientific outcome measurement.

Looking to the USA for answers

In this book we have tried to develop an international approach to some of the health regulatory issues discussed and to this end we have a chapter which looks at the tort systems and clinical negligence in the USA.

We have done this because regulators of health care and health quality in the UK often look to the USA for ideas. Health quality management improvement tools such as clinical guidelines and practice parameters are prime examples of this. The USA is seen by many as the cradle of clinical risk management.

Taking all the above into account, it is worrying to read from US news reports that all is not well in certain areas of US health and health quality regulation. This all raises the uncomfortable question that if matters are not going well in the USA, then what hope is there for the NHS, which has far less developed healthcare quality management programmes, which are an essential feature of any health regulation process.

Boodman in the Washington Post[3] states that not much has changed structurally in the USA to make healthcare treatment safer for patients. This is despite the widely publicised IOM (Institute of Medicine) Report[4], *To Err is Human*, which shocked the nation.

US medical malpractice crisis

There is also a medical malpractice crisis currently playing out in the USA on a scale causing alarm and despondency to many health carers. Many health carers would argue that the UK is also facing a clinical malpractice crisis.

It is important to examine the reasons for the USA clinical negligence crisis as there may be lessons that we can learn and use to help us understand our own problems. There is also the need to be aware of the dangers of comparing the US problems with the UK, as can happen in arguments and policy debates over the direction of UK health policy regulation. The US litigation crisis could be held up as an example of what can happen with an non-reformed tort system. The validity of citing US problems in the UK does need to be questioned.

Differing problems

The scale of the US problems and the general responses to them are interesting, but they are essentially different from those in the UK. In the USA, doctors are going on strike over the amount that they have to pay for professional indemnity insurance cover as more of them are being sued for malpractice. Doctors have been striking in West Virginia, New Jersey and Pennsylvania to protest at the soaring costs of malpractice insurance premiums.[5] Healthcare providers in states without reasonable limits on non-economic damages have experienced the largest increases in premiums – between 36% and 113%, in 2002. These greatly increased costs are threatening access to health care, as doctors leave their practices and move to states that have enacted medical liability reforms.[6] The state of Nevada is facing unprecedented problems in assuring access to urgently needed care and a hospital had to close a trauma centre for 10 days because its surgeons quit as they could no longer afford malpractice insurance. Doctors are also retiring early or reducing their practice to patients who present less of a risk of litigation.[7] President Bush is calling for urgent reforms. 'There are too many lawsuits in America, and there are too many lawsuits filed against doctors and hospitals without merit'.[5]

President Bush[6] proposes that the US Congress take action to remedy the problem and suggested measures include:

- Ensure that old cases cannot be brought years after an event.
- Provide for payments of judgments over time rather than in a single lump sum.
- Reserve punitive damages for cases where they are justified.
- Ensure that recoveries for non-economic damages do not exceed a reasonable amount (US$250 000).

Is it also happening here in the UK?

We also have record levels of clinical negligence litigation in the UK[8] and calls have been made for a no-fault based liability system and that issue is discussed by our contributors. The NHS currently has potential liabilities for clinical negligence of £5.25 billion at 31 March 2002.[9] But are we really facing a similar situation to the USA? Has the American litigation tide swept across the Atlantic or is it already here? Will our doctors go on strike over litigation?

Clinical negligence litigation is a problem in the UK

We should not pretend that clinical negligence litigation is not a problem in the UK; it is, but not to the same extent as it is in the USA. To many, our clinical negligence litigation system is inefficient, expensive, slow, cumbersome and does not always produce the right remedy for the patient. It gives monetary damages but patients do not always need or want cash. They may seek a change in their care regime, an explanation and an apology of what went wrong. Money can never really adequately compensate for the loss of a faculty or amenity or a loved one.

The Chief Medical Officer's review of clinical negligence in the NHS has been published and is discussed in Chapter 4. There will no doubt be changes to our system, but it is important to maintain a sense of perspective. We are far from the extent of the problems in the USA and are never likely to reach that level – we are essentially different.

The difference

Americans spend proportionately far more per person on the costs of litigation than any other country in the world.[7] Unlike England, where judges award compensation, in the USA, juries award compensation and multi-million dollar awards are commonplace. In England, judges are notoriously conservative in their damages awards. As the jury awards go up so do insurance premiums. Lawyers in the USA, unlike the UK, operate on a contingency fee, which enables them to take a percentage of the damages award.

For English hospital doctors, unlike their USA counterparts, medical malpractice insurance premiums are not an issue. They are covered for clinical negligence malpractice by the CNST (Clinical Negligence Scheme for Trusts) which is an NHS scheme, managed and administered by the NHSLA (National Health Service Litigation Authority).[10]

A confident future?

There is every room for confidence in the expectation that these levels will fall as the NHS learns how better to control clinical risks and report errors. The National Patient Safety Agency (NPSA)[11] programmes have the potential to make a real difference to patient safety. The USA clinical malpractice crisis should not be seen to influence the clinical negligence policy makers in the UK, as to do so would fail to take into account the number of fundamental differences that exist between the systems.

The reform of health regulation systems and that of improving the quality of health care are issues that are going to be with us for some time. The chapters in this book show that there are no easy solutions to the many problems that can be seen to exist in the area.

John Tingle
Reader in Health Law
Nottingham Law School
The Nottingham Trent University

References

1 CHI (Commission for Health Improvement). Getting Better? A Report on the NHS. London: The Stationery Office; 2003.
2 CHI (Commission for Health Improvement). South North Divide in the NHS, News Release, 27 November 2002, London: CHI; 2002. Online. Available: www.chi.nhs.uk/eng/news/2002/nov/21.shtml
3 Boodman SG. No end to errors. Washington Post, 3 December 2002:HE01.
4 IOM (Institute of Medicine). To err is human, building a safer health system. In: Kohn LT, Corrigan JM, Donaldson MS, eds. Committee on Quality of Health Care in America. Washington, DC: National Academy Press; 2000.
5 Watson. Bush takes action against 'junk' medical lawsuits. The Times, 17 January 2003.
6 White House. Office of the Press Secretary: President calls for medical liability reform. Press release, 16 January 2003. Online. Available: http://www.whitehouse.gov/news/releases/2003/01/print/20030116.html
7 US Department of Health and Human Services. Confronting the new health care crisis: improving health care quality and lowering costs by fixing our medical liability system. Washington, DC: Office of the Assistant Secretary for Planning and Evaluation; 24 July 2002.
8 NAO. Handling clinical negligence claims in England, HC 403. London: The Stationery Office; May 2001. Online. Available: www.nao.gov.uk
9 NAO. NHS (England) Summarised Accounts 2001–2002, HC 493 2002–2003. London: The Stationery Office; 2003.
10 NHSLA (National Health Service Litigation Authority). The NHSLA Publications website; 2003. Online. Available: http://www.nhsla.com
11 NPSA (The National Patient Safety Agency). Frequently asked questions. London: NPSA; May 2003. Online. Available: http://www.npsa.nhs.uk/

Chapter 1

Clinical governance: a means for improving and regulating quality

Keith Haynes

THE CONTEXT: THE EMERGENCE OF CLINICAL GOVERNANCE

When the Labour administration came to power in May 1997, its first published White Paper on health, *The New NHS; Modern, Dependable*, set out its plans for the NHS, centring on quality and performance issues. To achieve this, the government set out six key principles for the modern NHS (Box 1.1). The White Paper explicitly stated[1] that:

'The government will require every NHS trust to embrace the concept of clinical governance, so that quality is at the core, both of their responsibilities as organisations, and of each of their staff as individual professionals.'

It describes clinical governance, specifically as:

'A system which is able to demonstrate, in both primary and secondary care, that systems are in place guaranteeing clinical quality improvements at all levels of healthcare provision. Healthcare organisations will be accountable for the quality of services they provide.'

> **Box 1.1   Six key principles of the modern NHS**
>
> 1 To re-establish the NHS as a national service for all patients throughout the country where patients will receive high quality care regardless of age, gender or culture if they are ill or injured.
> 2 To establish national standards based upon best practices, which will be influenced and delivered locally by the healthcare professionals themselves taking into account the needs of the local population.
> 3 Collaborative working partnerships between hospital, community services and local authorities, where the patient is the central focus.
> 4 Ensuring that the services are delivering high quality care and providing value for money.
> 5 To establish an internal culture where clinical quality is guaranteed for all.
> 6 To enhance public confidence in the NHS.
>
> *Source*: Department of Health, 1997.[1]

This duty was then enshrined in the Health Act 1999 (s.18) as follows:

'It is the duty of each health authority, primary care trust and NHS trust to put and keep in place arrangements for the purpose of monitoring and improving the quality of health care which it provides to individuals.'

This legal requirement is delivered through the various components of clinical governance set out below.

In 1998, the quality reforms were described in some detail in the consultation document[2] *A First Class Service: Quality in the NHS*. This outlined the creation of new national agencies such as the National Institute for Clinical Excellence and the Commission for Health Improvement. Importantly, it set out a definition for clinical governance as follows:

'A framework through which NHS organisations are accountable for continuously improving the quality of their services, and safeguarding high standards of care by creating an environment in which excellence in clinical care will flourish.'

A summary of the key components of these quality reforms is set out in Box 1.2. Clinical governance is perceived as the 'lynchpin' behind quality improvement in the NHS.

We should be clear, however, that the origin of clinical governance is unmistakably political and is rooted very much in the events of the period. There had been a series of major quality failures in areas such as paediatric cardiac surgery, cervical screening, histology reporting and gynaecological treatment, which had been widely reported.[3] As a consequence the government found itself responding to a loss of public confidence in health professionals and the need for a system which demonstrated the accountability of health professionals.

Box 1.2   Summary of the key components of NHS quality reforms

Clinical governance
A new statutory responsibility for NHS organisations and those who lead them to put in place a framework for quality improvement, in which high standards are safeguarded, continuous improvement is promoted and excellence is encouraged.

National service frameworks
Nationally developed guidance on service planning and delivery for major care areas or patient groups, which provides a template or model against which services locally can be benchmarked and which can be used to promote changes where they are needed.

National framework for assessing performance
A six dimensional framework for performance improvement – health improvement, access, effectiveness, efficiency, patient experience, health outcomes. To be used in existing performance review and in new initiatives (such as national service frameworks) as a structure for measurement. Also used in the development of new sets of published clinical indicators.

National patient safety and user survey
A regular national survey of patients' and users' experience of the NHS, providing comparative information on patients' views.

National Institute for Clinical Excellence
A new national centre for appraising the clinical and cost effectiveness of healthcare interventions, which issues authoritative guidance to the NHS on the use of such interventions.

Commission for Health Improvement
A new national organisation responsible for monitoring and reporting on the arrangements for clinical governance in NHS organisations, for providing national leadership in clinical governance, and for investigating and intervening when particular problems or failures are identified, including supporting and assisting with formal inquiries.

Source: Department of Health, 1998.[2]

In light of the various scandals, concerns emerged in the mind of politicians and the public about the arrangements for self-regulation of the medical profession, the existence of a protective and closed culture in some NHS organisations and the apparent failure of the medical profession and managers in these organisations to deal with, in some cases, longstanding quality issues.

To some extent, clinical governance was a concept waiting to be invented. It very easily evolved out of the corporate governance initiatives of the government, which had been in response to scandals in the corporate investment world. Following the publication of the Cadbury Report[4] in 1992 the NHS developed its own principles of corporate governance which are contained in *Corporate Governance in the NHS: Code of Conduct and Code of Accountability*.[5] Not surprisingly, following the introduction of the concept and the imposition of a quality imperative the General Medical Council has reported an increase in the number of referrals to it.[6]

'Clinical governance' therefore has been the convenient banner to enable politicians to demonstrate to the public, accountability of the medical profession.

CLINICAL GOVERNANCE: DEFINING THE INDEFINABLE

Clinical governance has been defined[2] as: 'A framework through which NHS organisations are accountable for continuously improving the quality of their services and safeguarding high standards of care by creating an environment in which excellence in clinical care will flourish.'

However, trying to define clinical governance in terms that are meaningful to the healthcare professional at the coalface, and that are consistently understood, is much more difficult. Although a clear vision has been articulated by some commentators,[7,8] others have argued that it is much more difficult to turn the vision into reality.[9,10] Referring to the Donaldson and Scally[8] article, Goodman[9] observes that 'the essay is all thought and no action, an epitome of hope over expectation, a high clarion call of wonderful things just over the horizon'. In primary care, it has been described as an 'all encompassing', 'elastic' and 'chaotic' theoretical concept, with something of a 'vast amoeba' about it, which requires considerable effort to produce a workable definition.[11]

Agreeing on a meaningful definition of 'clinical governance' that is of value to practitioners makes it difficult to regulate and inspect quality within healthcare organisations, which is the role that falls to the Commission for Health Improvement. However there have been attempts[12] to give the concept a more meaningful and useful definition as 'the means by which organisations ensure the provision of quality clinical care by making individuals accountable for setting, maintaining and monitoring performance standards'.

Donaldson and Scally[8] recognise that historically quality was seen as something that was inherent in the system, sustained by the ethos and skills of the health professionals working within the organisation. The North Thames Department of Public Health discussion paper[12] suggests that the concept of clinical governance moves this relationship between the organisation and individual practitioner onto an altogether different level. The consequence of clinical governance is that in healthcare organisations both the individual and the institution have separate and complementary responsibilities for ensuring the quality of clinical care. It notes that the 'crucial difference now is that because standard setting is becoming mandatory, institutional support is no longer discretionary. Now the institution is required to ensure that appropriate standards are set and maintained by all their clinicians. This involves a shift from a passive to an active involvement of the institution'. This is the real difference that clinical governance has brought. Management has a real responsibility to empower clinicians at the coalface to help them feel more responsible for providing quality care, making management a very active partner in the delivery of the quality component of care. Latham et al.[13] concur with the view that clinical governance as an initiative to improve quality is very different from the approaches that have gone before because it is underpinned by a new statutory duty of quality.

Donaldson and Scally[8] set out a definition of clinical governance that has been promoted by the Clinical Governance Support Unit and more importantly the Commission for Health Improvement. The key components of clinical governance that are identified in this model are:

- Consultation and patient involvement
- Clinical audit
- Clinical risk management
- Research and effectiveness
- Staffing and staff management
- Education, training and continuing professional and personal development
- Use of information to support clinical governance and healthcare delivery.

Although these are the broad headings, it is less clear what makes up the ingredients under each of these headings that lead to effective clinical governance. Nevertheless these are the headings which the Commission for Health Improvement use when carrying out their reviews of NHS organisations.

To be effective, a clinical governance programme must include the following key dimensions (Figure 1.1):

- A process for recording and deriving lessons from untoward incidents, complaints and claims
- A risk management programme

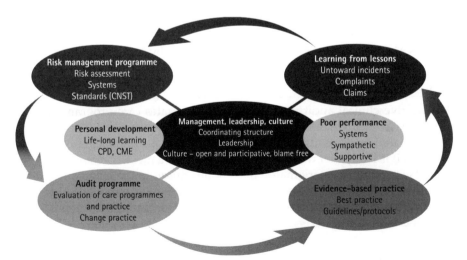

Figure 1.1   Dimensions of clinical governance in practice. (©Reproduced with permission from Haynes edition 12 of Casebook – the Journal for Members of the Medical Protection Society.)

- Effective clinical audit
- Evidence-based medical practice
- A supportive, non-blaming culture committed to the concept of life-long learning.

Introduced in isolation, none of these dimensions will provide effective clinical governance. The key is to ensure they are connected and that the loop is closed, thereby providing a coherent and comprehensive programme. Success in achieving this will depend on strong and effective management and leadership whose primary aim is to foster an open and participative 'fair blame' culture that emphasises both avoiding and learning from mistakes in equal measure.

Learning from experience

Healthcare organisations, but especially NHS trusts, have available to them a rich source of material generated by untoward incident reporting, complaints and claims, but sometimes this information is not put to good use. Often the completion of an untoward incident report or the final letter to a complainant are seen as ends in themselves. Taking the process a stage further, however, by using the material to identify changes that need to be made may require minimal effort. What is needed is a multidisciplinary mechanism for reporting and systematically reviewing untoward incidents, complaints and claims to distil the lessons that can be learned from them. The need for NHS organisations to achieve this objective became a key recommendation of the Chief Medical Officer's landmark report *An Organisation with a Memory*.[14]

Risk management programme

Healthcare organisations need to ensure that they have in place effective risk management systems and programmes based on a paper assessment of clinical risk and with appropriate controls to manage the risk.

Clinical audit programme

An effective clinical audit programme that evaluates care programmes and practice is also an essential component of clinical governance. It should also be able to demonstrate that practice has changed as a consequence of the programme. It is likely that where clinical audit is being most effectively used the subjects for audit have originated from issues raised in the risk management programme, or are being used to test evidence-based practice. To be most effective the clinical audit programme should reflect key organisational issues and concerns.

Evidence-based practice

Recent incidents have demonstrated that clinicians can differ widely in their perceptions of current and best practice. A key issue for health organisations is to know what is current best practice and to know that this is being practised within the organisation.

Management, leadership and culture

The critical and cohesive element of a successful clinical governance programme is effective management and leadership that fosters a real cultural change. This will only be achieved through an open and participative 'fair blame' culture. An essential ingredient is a commitment to the concepts of life-long learning and professional development.

THE REGULATORY FRAMEWORK FOR THE IMPLEMENTATION OF CLINICAL GOVERNANCE: COMMISSION FOR HEALTH IMPROVEMENT

The Commission for Health Improvement (CHI) was set up to improve the quality of patient care in the NHS in England and Wales. It started operating from 1 April 2000 and conducts clinical governance reviews of NHS acute and specialist trusts, mental health trusts, NHS Direct sites, ambulance trusts, primary care trusts in England and local health groups in Wales. CHI also investigates serious service failures in the NHS. Investigations can be triggered by concerns originating in CHI or by a request from the Secretary of State for Health in England or the Welsh Assembly government. Since its inception it has already carried out a large number of reviews in NHS organisations and some special investigations.[15]

The Prime Minister, Tony Blair, has described CHI's creation as the 'boldest step yet' in the drive to modernise the NHS.

It has also been described as the fastest growing institution in the NHS, doubling its budget from £12m in 2000/01 to £25m in 2002/03, increasing its staff from 180 to 300 and the number of part-time reviewers to 500.[16]

CHI's current roles are to:

- Monitor and help improve the quality of NHS patient care through a rolling programme of reviews of arrangements for clinical governance in all NHS bodies:
  - In support of this during 2001/02, CHI carried out and published 102 clinical governance reviews.[15] It is due to visit every NHS organisation in England and Wales on a rolling programme.
- Investigate serious service failures:
  - CHI also investigates serious service failures when requested by the Secretary of State for Health in England or the National Assembly for Wales, although it can do so at the request of NHS organisations and as a result of their own clinical governance reviews.
- Review progress with the implementation of national standards set by National Institute for Clinical Excellence guidance, National Service Frameworks and other NHS priorities:
  - In conjunction with the Audit Commission, CHI has already carried out the first in a series of national studies measuring the implementation of

all national service frameworks across the NHS, resulting in a report into NHS cancer care in England and Wales.
- Provide advice and guidance on the implementation of clinical governance:
  - As part of its review process and the publication of its reports, CHI has a leading role to play in disseminating best practice.

CHI has identified six core principles that guide its work[15]:

1 CHI will put the patient experience at the centre of its work. It seeks to capture patient views so that NHS staff can appreciate how their services are being experienced, particularly by those who may have difficulty in accessing services.
2 CHI will be independent, rigorous and fair. Here CHI is keen to emphasise that it is independent of government and that its assessments will be thorough. It will highlight areas of excellence but will not hold back from pointing out where there are areas for improvement.
3 CHI will have a role that is developmental and support the NHS in its efforts to improve continuously.
4 CHI's work will be based on the best available evidence and focus on improvement.
5 CHI will be open and will strive continuously to improve accessibility of its work and findings. To this end all of its reviews and publications are available on its website (http://www.chi.gov.uk/).
6 CHI will apply the same standards of continuous improvement to itself that it expects of others. Interestingly, in its early days, CHI commissioned a joint report with the NHS Confederation about its review process, as a result of which changes were made.

However, its role and functions are set to change and grow considerably following the NHS Reform and Healthcare Professions Act 2002.[17] A new Commission for Healthcare Audit and Inspection (CHAI) will be created from April 2004 in England and Wales to include the current role and functions of CHI as well as the following new responsibilities:

- All of the current and proposed work of the Commission for Health Improvement
- National NHS value for money work for the Audit Commission
- Independent healthcare work of the National Care Standards Commission.

When the relevant provisions of the NHS Reform and Healthcare Professions Act 2002 are commenced, CHI will also have to:

- inspect NHS organisations and services
- carry out independent performance assessments of annual comparative NHS performance ratings in England (including star ratings of NHS trusts), commissioning of national clinical audits, and management of annual staff and patient surveys in England
- recommend the government takes special measures where it finds NHS services are of unacceptably poor quality or there are serious failings in the way they are being run

- publish an annual report to parliament and the National Assembly for Wales on the state of services to NHS patients.

The background to this significant change is the recognition by government that in the area of regulation and inspection, there are overlaps between the existing bodies. In its Statement of Purpose[18] on the role of the new CHAI it acknowledges that the current overlaps cause unnecessary burdens on front line staff who are faced with the need to respond to uncoordinated inspections, audits and reviews. The Statement of Purpose goes on to explain the underlying purpose for the establishment of one health and one social care inspectorate (the Commission for Social Care Inspection – CSCI) is so that:

- 'patients and service users will have clear assurances about the safety and quality and efficiency of the services they receive
- the burden of regulation on providers of health and social care services will be reduced when services improve
- taxpayers will be assured that public funds are being used effectively
- the impact of inspection in generating better quality health and care services will be increased'.

The Statement of Purpose makes it clear that CHAI will be an independent body, established as a non-departmental body, acting at arm's length from government. The chair and commissioners of both bodies will be appointed through an independent process and not by the Secretary of State and these will in turn appoint the chief executive. The independence of the new body will be underpinned by a requirement to publish its findings and to report annually to parliament. The key functions of CHAI are set out in Box 1.3.

Box 1.3   Key functions of the Commission for Healthcare Audit and Inspection[18]

1 In accordance with national standards and service priorities, CHAI will inspect the management, provision and quality of health care. For the first time, the inspection of both public and private health care will be carried out by a single body. CHAI will also track where, and how well, public resources are being used so that not only the quality but also the value for money of services will be examined by a single inspectorate.
2 CHAI will carry out investigations into serious service failures, reporting to the public on what has happened, why, and how a repetition might be avoided. It will play a key role in identifying lessons to be learnt.
3 Whenever they have serious concerns about the quality of public services or the way in which they are being run, CHAI will be obliged to report this to the Secretary of State, with the ability to recommend that steps are taken to secure improvements in services.

4 CHAI will publish annual performance ratings, taking account of national priorities, for all NHS organisations in England. It will also produce annual reports to parliament on the state of health care. These independent assessments will play a key role in strengthening public accountability.

5 CHAI will collaborate with the Commission for Social Care Inspection (CSCI) to ensure joint approaches to integrated services. It will also help to coordinate the activity of other relevant review and inspection bodies. It is acknowledged that this will be particularly important, as there is a need for better coordination between the variety of bodies with inspection roles.

6 CHAI will carry out an independent review function for NHS complaints in England. It is agreed that placing this responsibility within CHAI will provide the necessary independence and speedier resolution of complaints, as well as a direct link into quality improvement processes.

7 CHAI will register, inspect and regulate providers in the independent sector against national minimum standards. Where it finds that the quality of provision falls substantially below these standards, particularly where the safety or welfare of service users is at risk, they will be able to take enforcement action and, if serious concerns persist, to remove the provider's registration.

CHAI will also:

8 Inspect clinical governance arrangements that local NHS organisations have in place to ensure effective quality assurance and quality improvement.

9 Ensure appropriate arrangements are in place to promote public health.

10 Carry out any national healthcare studies covering both England and Wales.

11 Inspect NHS foundation trusts and report on its findings to an independent regulator, who will be responsible for their regulation. CHAI may also recommend that the independent regulator take special measures where it has serious concerns about the quality of services provided.

12 Replace the Mental Health Act Commission in providing enhanced scrutiny of the operation of compulsion under the new Mental Health Bill.

Source: CHAI, 2003.[18]

THE IMPACT OF CLINICAL GOVERNANCE AND ITS REGULATION

While the government acknowledges that the current arrangements for the regulation of health care and, in particular its quality, may not be working as well as they would wish[18] and are about to strengthen the arrangements with the creation of CHAI, it is timely to reflect upon the impact of clinical governance to date.

What has CHI as the regulatory body itself said about the implementation and impact of clinical governance to date? CHI itself has noted that there are a number of emerging causes for concern[15]:

● Organisation-wide policies and strategies regarding clinical governance are not being formulated.

- Policies and strategies not being implemented. CHI observes that there are instances of policies and strategies not being implemented or being implemented partially or ineffectively across every area of clinical governance activity.
- A tendency for organisations to be reactive rather than proactive. CHI notes that this theme emerged where organisations did not anticipate problems and threats to quality, responding only to those causing particular, often public, concerns.
- Not sharing learning across and between organisations. Where good practice was identified as a result of a clinical governance review CHI feel that this is not being shared.
- A failure to communicate from strategic to operational level, particularly on the part of boards and clinical leaders to share their vision, values and policies.
- The existence of barriers to communication between disciplines and staff groups within clinical areas. CHI identified that this is a persistent theme, which it feels undermines the effective delivery of health care.

More importantly, CHI has identified[15] that four of the seven components of their definition of clinical governance stand out as a cause for concern, identified as follows:

- Risk management
- Staffing and staff management
- Patient involvement
- Use of information.

Dealing with risk management specifically, it is very interesting that despite the fact that risk as a discipline has been around for some time[19,20] and is a key element of clinical governance, CHI has still found that trusts are poor at managing risks to patients and, in particular, having in place effective adverse event reporting systems which staff are trained in the use of and are signed up to using. Often cited as a reason for healthcare staff not reporting adverse incidents[21] is the fear of blame and retribution, underpinning the reality that clinical governance is as much about creating the right culture in organisations as having in place systems. If risk management is to be taken as a measure of the success of clinical governance then there is clearly some way to go (see Boxes 1.4 and 1.5: Risk management lessons in secondary and primary care: *Source* CHI reports).

A survey of all 47 trusts in the West Midlands[13] found that clinical governance had not been advanced beyond the production of strategies, establishing committees and appointing leads. In particular there was little evidence of the cultural change that clinical governance requires and that the concept still had to make a real difference at the clinical workface. It acknowledged that this is easier to say than do and that previous efforts to mandate the development of quality improvement structures and processes in healthcare organisations, through central directives and initiatives, have not been particularly successful either in the UK or other countries.[22]

Box 1.4 Extracts from CHI reports: Risk management lessons in secondary care

Question

How well do the trust and the staff anticipate things that might go wrong? Does the trust encourage staff to report problems? Does it have systematic methods for collecting information about risks to patients? Does it have systems for making sure managers and staff learn from mistakes?

Answer: Trust 1

A new risk management system was introduced and seems to be working well. Most staff have embraced the process for reporting incidents but doctors are still reluctant to do so ... Some areas have had risk assessments carried out but the trust needs to develop a routine risk assessment programme for all areas.

Answer: Trust 2

The trust has a well-established single incident reporting system. Staff have a good awareness of the system and how to use it. However staff knowledge and understanding of the importance of near misses is poor. Information from risks or mistakes is not always fed back to staff or acted upon, although CHI found pockets of good practice.

Source: CHI reports sourced from http://www.chi.org.uk

Box 1.5 Extracts from CHI pilot reviews of PCTs: Developing as a learning organisation

'CHI found little evidence of formal learning mechanisms for PCT employed staff in areas such as reported incidents. [The PCT should consider developing] a clinical risk management system that facilitates the management and monitoring of incidents and how to learn from them.'
(Central Manchester PCT: CHI clinical governance review, p. 7)

'The [PCT] should build on the success of reporting systems for significant events in primary care so it has a comprehensive overview of the risks it faces in the services it provides.'
(Fenland PCT: CHI clinical governance review, p. 4)

CHI expects the PCT to 'increase awareness of risk management policies, extend the system of incident reporting across all staff groups and develop a system for near miss reporting.'
(Hillingdon PCT and NHS Direct West London: CHI clinical governance review, p. 4)

Source: CHI reports sourced from http://www.chi.org.uk

In primary care, although clinical governance is welcomed as a positive and long overdue process, it has been found to be a challenge to implement.[23] A shortage of funding, a lack of guidance and a concern over the speed of implementation and the volume of work are identified as having hampered progress. Many of those involved in the study[23] saw clinical governance as a process to be embedded over a number of years and had adopted a gentle and facilitative approach to their role and the practices they worked with, recognising it as a long game. Many of the conclusions and recommendations from this study (Box 1.6) only serve to corroborate that the implementation of successful clinical governance relies upon effective leadership skills.[13,24] Disappointingly Latham et al.[13] were not convinced that those leading clinical governance in trusts were investing sufficient time and energy to translating their personal commitment to the concept into organisational action.

Box 1.6   Conclusions and recommendations from the study of the introduction of clinical governance in primary care in the South West of England

At the PCG level
- It is critical for the continuing development of the process that GPs remain engaged and inspired by clinical governance and engage other colleagues across the PCG.
- A clear understanding of the responsibilities inherent in the role of the clinical governance lead would facilitate the selection process and provide focus for the lead and other members of the PCG.
- PCG clinical governance leads may benefit from explicit guidelines on the 'carrots and sticks' that they may use, and of the associated consequences of non-compliance.
- Adequate financial resources should be set aside for clinical governance leads to be able to do the job properly.
- A multi-professional clinical governance team approach is likely to be the most sustainable model.
- Nurses, midwives, health visitors and managers should be encouraged to play a role in developing clinical governance.

At the practice level
- Clinical governance leads should continue to use a supportive and facilitative approach to implementation.
- Ownership of the process can be facilitated by encouraging time for reflection and providing adequate financial resources for protected time, training and dissemination of information at a practice level.
- Practices need to begin to see some tangible outcomes as a result of the efforts invested in clinical governance.

Source: Sweeney CM, Sweeney KG, Greco MJ, Stead JW. Moving clinical governance forward: capturing the experiences of primary care group leads. Clinical Governance Bulletin 2001; 2(1):April.

The National Audit Office study, *Achieving Improvements through Clinical Governance: A Progress Report on Implementation by NHS Trusts*, concluded that, while the structures and organisational arrangements to make clinical governance happen were in place, progress in implementing clinical governance is patchy, varying between trusts, within trusts and between the components of clinical governance.[25] Although acknowledging that clinical governance had brought a range of achievements including clinical quality issues being more mainstream, a greater and more explicit accountability of both clinicians and managers, and more transparent and collaborative working, most trusts still viewed clinical governance in terms of structures and process. The study concluded that although most of the components that make up clinical governance and which predated the introduction of the concept in 1999 are in place, the coverage of each component within individual trusts varies from those with less than 20% to ones with over 80% coverage. It observes that although medical audit as a discipline has been around for 14 years, it remains underdeveloped in many trusts. Risk management fares better, with an acknowledgement that it has developed substantially since 1999. Despite this, in 17% of trusts, the proportion of clinical directorates using clinical risk management is still 60% or below. Furthermore, although trusts have improved the recording, collating and review of data, training in risk management is still weak as is the performance in taking action on those risks that have been identified. Progress therefore seems to be a bit like the curate's egg but overall it seems that there is a clear need to do better.

Given what has been described as the 'vast amoeba'-like[11] qualities of the definition of the concept of clinical governance, a real difficulty lies in knowing that it works and being able to measure its progress.[13] Latham et al.[13] recognised that there is an urgent need for good measures of progress in clinical governance which are based on assessments by other stakeholders and data gathered from people working directly within an organisation. This is what CHI has been seeking to achieve although with some criticism of a lack of consistency in its reporting.[16]

The US experience seems no better. You might have thought that in a nation that has had regulation for some time that improved standards, better quality and improved patient safety might have been the outcome. A recent article in the *Washington Post*[26] has identified that 3 years after a landmark report found pervasive medical mistakes in American hospitals, little has been done to reduce death and injury. It acknowledges that the Institute of Medicine's report *To Err is Human*[27] was greeted with a flurry of activity. Congress held hearings, earmarked US$50m for research into the causes and presentation of medical mistakes, and gained President Clinton's support for mandatory reporting of serious incidents.

The report says that there is a lot of talk but no significant progress which is attributed to the opposition of doctors and hospitals to mandatory reporting, a lack of oversight by the Federal government and the absence of an effective lobby. One observer comments that the incessant talk about safety and the lack of concrete action 'illustrates the difference between meeting-room reality and in-the-theatres reality'.

Potentially, this does not augur well for the future of the concept of clinical governance. While CHI and other commentators have highlighted good practice as a consequence of clinical governance, there is clearly a long way to go. The new Commission for Healthcare Audit and Inspection would do well to offer a more helpful and more meaningful definition of the concept of clinical governance and a robust framework for assessing its contribution and success. Only with these two components in place are we likely to know that clinical governance makes a difference.

References

1 Department of Health. The new NHS: modern, dependable. London: The Stationery Office; 1997.

2 Department of Health. A first class service: quality in the new NHS. London: The Stationery Office; 1998.

3 Smith R. All changed, changed utterly. British medicine will be transformed by the Bristol case. British Medical Journal 1998; 316(7149):1917–1918.

4 Committee on the Financial Aspects of Corporate Governance (The Cadbury Report). London: Gee; 1992.

5 Department of Health. Corporate governance in the NHS, code of conduct, code of accountability. London: HMSO; 1994.

6 Hospital Doctor, GMC complaints, 9 January 2003:3; Doctor, GMC complaints, 9 January 2003:15.

7 Donaldson LJ, Muir Gray JA. Clinical governance: a quality duty for health organisations. Quality in Health Care 1998; 7(Suppl):37–44.

8 Donaldson LJ, Scally G. Clinical governance and the drive for quality improvement in the new NHS in England. British Medical Journal 1998; 317:61–65.

9 Goodman NW. Clinical governance. British Medical Journal 1998; 317(7174):1725–1727.

10 Goodman NW. Accountability, clinical governance and the acceptance of imperfection. Journal of the Royal Society of Medicine 2000; 93(2):56–58.

11 Sweeney G, Stead J, Sweeney K, Greco M. Exploring the implementation and development of clinical governance in primary care within the South West Region: views from PCG clinical governance leads. The Wisdom Centre; 2000. Online. Available: http://www.wisdomnet.co.uk/sweeney.htm

12 NHSE North Thames Region Office, Department of Public Health. Clinical Governance in North Thames. A paper for discussion and consultation. NHSE; 1998.

13 Latham L, Freeman T, Walshe K, et al. Clinical governance: from policy to practice. University of Birmingham: Health Services Management Centre; 2000.

14 Department of Health. An organisation with a memory. Report of an expert group on learning from adverse events in the NHS. London: The Stationery Office; 2000.

15 CHI's combined annual report and accounts 2001–2002. Growing a new organisation. Online. Available: http://www.chi.gov.uk

16 Day P, Klein R. Who nose best? Health Service Journal, 4 April 2002.

17 NHS Reform and Healthcare Professions Act 2002. London: The Stationery Office; 2002.

18 Commission for Healthcare Audit and Inspection and the Commission for Social Care Inspection, Statement of Purpose; 2003. Online. Available: www.doh.gov.uk/statementofpurpose/index.htm

19 NHSE. Risk Management in the NHS. London: HMSO; 1994.

20 NHS Litigation Authority. Clinical Negligence Scheme for Trusts: Clinical risk management standards. June 2002.

21 Nicklin PJ. Perceptions and attitudes towards Clinical Risk, the findings of a stakeholder survey 2001 (unpublished). Medical Protection Society and University of York.

22 Walshe K (ed.). Evaluating clinical audit: past lessons, future directions. London: Royal Society of Medicine; 1995.

23 Sweeney CM, Sweeney KG, Greco MJ, Stead JW. Softly, softly, the way forward? A qualitative study of the first year of implementing clinical governance in primary care. Primary Health Care Research & Development 2002; 3:53–65.

24 Sweeney CM, Sweeney KG, Greco MJ, Stead JW. Moving clinical governance forward: capturing the experiences of primary care group leads. Clinical Governance Bulletin 2001; 2(1):April.

25 National Audit Office. Work in progress: NHS – achieving improvements through clinical governance. London: National Audit Office; 2003. Online. Available: http://www.nao.gov.uk/publications/workinprogress/clinical_governance.htm

26 Boodman SG. No end to errors. Three years after a landmark report found pervasive medical mistakes in American hospitals, little has been done to reduce death or injury. *Washington Post*. Online. Available: www.washingtonpost.com/wp-dyn/articles/A58443-2002Nov30.html

27 The Institute of Medicine. To err is human. Washington, DC: National Academy Press; 2000. Online. Available: http://www.nap.edu/readingroom

Chapter 2

Health policy and provision: Public Management and its influence on regulation in England

Helen Caulfield

'Strong government regulation is also crucial ... regulations are required to ensure that quality standards are met, that financial fraud and other abuses do not take place, that those entitled to care are not denied services, and the confidentiality of medical information is respected.'[1]

'The regulation of the NHS in this broad sense must not, in our view, be in the day to day control of the Department of Health.'[2]

'where the NHS is decentralised with a plurality of providers operating within a framework of clear national standards regulated independently'[3]

INTRODUCTION

New Public Management is a relatively new theory of how governments can approach healthcare reform. It builds on academic thinking about the relative merits of governing through a monopolistic approach, a free market approach or a mix of elements of both in relation to public services. A central feature of this theory is that the government becomes a skilled administrator ensuring that other agencies provide the service, while the government remains in overall control of the regulation of those agencies as a means of ensuring that quality is maintained. The importance of regulation is that the government determines policy objectives followed by the creation of the structures needed to ensure implementation and enforcement of these policy objectives.

The UK has seen a discernible shift from its traditional monopolistic approach in ownership, manager and financier of the health service to a stronger emphasis on the role of state as administrator with other agencies owning, providing and managing the service. This approach allows for a much greater role for the private sector in the NHS. This shift has been balanced by a corresponding emphasis on regulation of quality and standard setting that is more national than local in nature.

This shift in regulatory emphasis is examined in England in relation to three main areas: people, settings and employers. Each of these is considered to determine how far the current government is adopting the regulatory components of New Public Management.

The main obstacle to the continued adoption of the theory of New Public Management is the diversity and power of the healthcare professional regulatory bodies. In order to achieve a state-based central administrative role in health, it is consistent with the theory of New Public Management that the staff must be regulated in similar fashion. The government's attempts to achieve this consistency are examined in relation to the creation of an overarching body for health professionals as well as the policy to promote the employer as the regulator of people within a framework of regulated settings.

The conclusion is that the government is actively decreasing the power of individual health professional regulators, while actively increasing regulation by the employer in direct relationship with the government.

NEW PUBLIC MANAGEMENT: CLASSIFICATION OF A THEORY IN HEALTH REFORM

Health system reform

Recent trends in thinking about the government's role in the health system have considered the extent to which functions of the health system should remain within the control of the government as well as the extent of that control. The functions are:

- policy
- service provision (promotion, prevention, cure)
- funding (taxation, social insurance)
- regulation (price, quality, quantity)
- resource allocation (agents to intermediaries).

Studies produce queries about whether there are factors or principles which can be replicated across more than one country,[1,4] with a growing realisation that money alone would not produce efficiency:

'for some services provided by the public sector, the system of provision is so grossly inefficient that it is unlikely to be cost effective no matter what interventions the system tries to provide. Such inefficiencies have been criticised so clearly and for so long that it is evident that they will only be overcome by radical changes in the organisation of health care: such as a shift in the government's role from providing care to financing care and stimulating competition among providers.'[1]

In developing countries, a desire to change policies previously developed as colonial legacies was further encouraged by economic crises which meant smaller budgets and less philanthropy. In developed nations, a desire to refocus government responsibility from traditional 'nation building' coincided with a perception of low system quality of services and user responsiveness. This trend continued in spite of the considerable variation in structures of health systems, population coverage, health benefits, and provision.[5]

Economic theory in health reform

Theories to explain why more affluent countries were failing in their provision or approach to health systems considered the economic approaches to health sectors. The theoretical underpinnings that have contributed to this perspective began from neoclassical economics, which asserts that intensive state intervention combined with ownership and control of the health sector is justified by problems of market failure:

- Externalities and public goods
- Imperfect information
- Risk and uncertainty
- Market structures.

There is no agreement about the extent to which these failures justify a large state role in any health system. There is more agreement that state intervention is justified to address the issues of equity and efficiency. This theory is not without problems; it points out the failures of the system without addressing the state's role or other structures that could be put in place to remedy the failures.[6]

Because this framework does not address the role of public ownership, it has led to the development of a new institutional economic theory. This provides a framework for understanding the effectiveness of different ownership and governance arrangements. This framework of economics of organisations groups together a variety of economic theories:

- *Principle–agent theory* which considers information, motivation and innovation. The contractual and governance arrangements developed under the competitive pressures of markets are applied to public sector organisations. On motivation for example, problems for health managers in determining outputs were regarded as 'inimical to the efficient management of the [sectors] concerned'.[7]
- *Transaction cost economics* which allows observation of the arrangements of activities within a hierarchy as opposed to interaction in a market with

suppliers or other contractors.[8] Research shows that a vertical hierarchy produces a weakening of incentives for productivity and that monopolies are maintained to protect low productivity state-owned enterprises from competition from more efficient producers.[9]

- *Public choice theory* where the domination of self-interest is a strong influence on the role of an organisation which in turn affects different incentive structures. This involves measuring how the incentives of politicians, interest groups and bureaucrats may affect behaviour in a way that creates rigid structures that reduce economic growth.[10]

New Public Management

New Public Management ideas embody a particular view on the nature of the state's role. The development of the theory of New Public Management was driven by a focus on managerial strategies that had the potential to lead to greater results from fewer resources. This theory also questioned the central planning adopted by a number of countries in the mid-twentieth century. Under this theory, the state should be involved in the policy, purchasing, regulation but not necessarily the provision of health care. This approach is more market orientated with an emphasis on the use of the private sector for the provision for public services.

> 'As governments move from a concern to do to a concern to ensure that things are done, the managerial focus has increasingly been directed away from formal process towards results ... These management innovations lead to the search for enhanced clarity of role and tighter lines of accountability with a desire to redefine the relationship between political policy making and administrative policy implementation.'[11]

New Public Management aims to improve the efficiency of provision of public services and its responsiveness to users. The means by which this is achieved are through the introduction of market mechanisms into public sector by the following:

- financial devolution and creation of autonomous executive agencies
- cost recovery
- use of explicit standards for assessing performance, with an emphasis on quality
- clear specification of relationships between inputs and outputs
- requirements for competitive tendering
- internal market arrangements.

New Public Management has been described as a means by which the state can justify accessing the private sector, and bringing its economic efficiencies into welfare provision.[12] This is a strong conceptual framework being applied in theory in both developed and developing countries. The core aim is to strengthen accountability of agents and to create incentives to bring the goals of the agent and the principle in closer alignment. This is achieved within a hierarchical structure where the objectives are clearly specified with a structure of incentives for good performance. New Public Management is a means for governments to move away from direct provision of health services to a more indirect role in regulating private providers and governing a managed market.[13] There is a greater emphasis on market activity management and the creation of policy rather than provision.

Some limitations of the theory of New Public Management are that the core assumptions may be inaccurate. Governments may not be more qualified at administration than they are at provision.[14] Large private sector corporations have similar problems to government organisations and may not automatically be better placed to deal with inefficiency in the system. Some academics caution against an approach that places the state in competition with the market.[15] Kaul points out that managerial pragmatism and political conviction are essential to motivate management innovation in government.[11] The transaction costs of decentralising central control to other providers may be significant and may be underestimated. Even where these obstacles are overcome, there is no guarantee that consumer choice will be strengthened and true consumer choice may remain weak.

The extent of success of this approach may not be seen for a number of years. In a study of health sector reforms of sub-Saharan Africa it became clear that the limited duration of many reforms and the limited nature of existing evaluation made it difficult to measure the effectiveness of the changes.[16]

HEALTH POLICY AND REGULATION

One of the key features of New Public Management involves the active management of regulatory frameworks where the role of government is to determine, impose and police such frameworks.[11] Regulation takes place when the state exerts control over the activities of individuals or firms[17] and in so doing takes action to manipulate prices, quantities and quality of products.[18] Regulation is provided by the state in response to the public demand for the correction of inefficient or inequitable market practices.[19] It is described as sustained and focused control exercised by a public agency over activities which are valued by the community.[20] Regulation is an inherently political process balancing the interests of different actors.[21]

The use of regulation has been described as a 'carrot and stick' approach where the state can influence the behaviour of private providers in health. Bennett et al.[22] set out five problems with private providers that can be overcome with regulatory mechanisms:

- a focus on maximising profit
- a failure to address public health
- lack of integration with government services
- attraction of health professionals out of the public sector
- provision of poor quality or inappropriate services.

Achieving the regulatory balance will depend on the level of economic development of the country, the strength of professional ethics, and the relative power of different interest groups. In this respect, the state and the private sector are motivated by different principles in their respective regard to regulatory structures. The state's influence in relation to regulation is directly related to its legislative power base, as well as power over resources and power over accountability and information. Major problems of regulation include professional self-interest, lack of information about who it is that needs to be regulated, and the government's organisational structure where regulation requires local responsibility and power.

The policy options available to a government in relation to regulation are to do nothing and allow for full competition, regulate where this costs time and effort, or to provide the services itself.[23] Bennett[24] proposes that the gap between those who advocate competition against those in favour of regulation may be less than both realise:

> 'In many ways the two approaches are complementary: regulation without consideration of the fundamentals of market structure and incentives is like treating the symptoms without addressing the cause.'

Kumaranayake[25] asserts that the main areas of regulation can be classified as:

- Entry: licensing, registration of facilities
- Prices: negotiation, rates of return
- Quality: certificate of need for new hospitals, patient protection
- Quantity: accreditation and use of registers
- Pharmaceuticals: for example, the World Trade Organisation prevents development of generic drugs.

The process of regulation can be classified as involving the following steps by the state:

- Setting the policy agenda
- Design and enactment of legislation
- Implementation
- Monitoring
- Enforcement and sanctioning.

In setting and designing regulation that fits the policy agenda, Kumaranayake[25] suggests that a number of key questions are addressed to assess why a form of regulation may be indicated:

- What are the state's policy objectives for desiring regulation?
- Is the policy aim to stop excess provision of medical care, contain costs or improve access to services?
- What is the problem preventing this policy objective from being reached?
- How does the existing structure fail to address this problem?
- What type of variable is to be regulated (for example, price, quality or quantity)?
- What are the mechanisms that have been used?

Factors critical to successful implementation include:

- information where lack of information is a problem for any regulator
- a strong central organisational structure with capacity to manage the regulatory process
- an estimation of the potentially significant transaction costs involved in the structure
- recognition that political influence and self-interest are necessary features of the structure
- clarity about who is responsible, how behaviour is monitored and what penalties exist
- institutional structures for the consumers and the regulator.

In developing countries, the main problem with regulatory structures is the ability of the state to ensure enforcement: this takes both capacity and skill on behalf of the state. Bennett[24] points out that 'one of the principal difficulties with regulation is that it requires substantial knowledge on the part of the regulatory body. In developed countries, governments have frequently found it difficult to acquire such information'. The use of incentive-based regulatory systems is considered to be more effective in developed countries where their role is not just to enforce minimum standards but also to have a positive influence on performance. This is beyond the capacity of many developing countries and can be very costly even for developed countries. Norton[26] considered incentives for nursing homes in the UK and found lower transaction costs existed when comparing incentive schemes with regulatory schemes. This did however rely on the need for constant monitoring and a sophisticated incentive design. The creation of Foundation Trusts in England is a form of incentive regulation designed to encourage hospitals to demonstrate efficiency in exchange for reduced regulatory control from the centre.

In England, it is clear that the Labour government is following a policy based on New Public Management. It appears that the policy objective is to achieve quality. In order to do so, quality needs to be measured and monitored. This is being achieved by the creation of regulatory structures taking on work previously carried out by the Department of Health, where standards of quality and performance are being developed and refined. The Secretary of State confirmed this policy direction:

'The Department of Health will focus on setting strategic objectives, determining standards, distributing and accounting for resources and securing the integrity of the overall system through for example, workforce planning and better IT. Overall the Department will be slimmed down as power and resources are devolved out of Whitehall. Some functions will move from the Department to the new Commission for Healthcare Audit and Inspection as the existing Commission for Health Improvement, National Care Standards Commission and the value for money work of the Audit Commission are brought together.'[27]

REGULATION OF INDIVIDUALS

The UK has eight regulatory bodies for health professionals. There are many health workers who are not regulated in such a formal manner, including healthcare assistants and all support staff who work to regulated professionals.

What characterises all of the existing regulatory bodies is that they have been established by statute at different times over the nineteenth and twentieth centuries. The bodies were all established on the principle of professional self-regulation with three main functions:

- Curriculum: to set standards of preparatory education for admission to the profession
- Conduct: to set standards for behaviour, and in some instances, competence
- Register: to create a current list of those who are able to practise in the profession.

Davies[28] describes professional self-regulation as:

'a legally protected monopoly or market shelter. In return for its privileged position, the profession makes an undertaking to act in the public interest. It will use its complex knowledge to set standards that work for the common good. It will also police its own members, removing from the register and hence prevent from practice those who fail to maintain those standards.'

Friedson[29] argued that a profession has gained a position in the division of labour that gives it autonomy and control over its own affairs. These members have achieved an 'extra-ordinary trustworthiness', by which they can be relied upon to put their knowledge and skills at the service of the public. The profession will ensure that each of their members maintains the ideals of practice and that newcomers are inducted in an appropriate way. The inherent risk is that this autonomy within regulation creates isolation. Davies[28] points out that this encourages the profession to see itself as the sole possessor of knowledge and virtue, to be somewhat suspicious of the technical and moral capacity of other occupations, and to be at best patronising and at worst contemptuous of its clientele.

This flaw in the process of regulation of individuals in the health sector has provoked criticism from powerful consumer groups. The National Consumer Council (NCC) commented that the position was 'a patchwork of varying arrangements for different professions, differences in regulation between public and independent sectors and legislation governing many regulatory bodies which has not caught up with changes in public demand or with current healthcare practices'.[30] The NCC's concerns focused on the vulnerable public and the difficulty for consumers of finding their way around the system. The NCC recommended better links between different types of regulation and consideration of a 'one-door' complaints system, more open business, and more participation of lay members.

A report from the Consumers Association[31] warned 'there is a danger that these changes will be reactive and fragmentary and will provide solutions to the problems of the last century, rather than to equip us to deal with the issues facing consumers and health care in this century'. Further criticism from Pyne[32] was that the interests being served by the regulatory bodies was inappropriate for the population served (Table 2.1).

The government is tackling this patchwork of regulation of health personnel in a concerted manner that acknowledges political constraints, particularly with doctors. The strategy began with the passing of Section 60 of the Health Act 1999. This first stage of reform allows the state to interfere with the legislative boundaries of each profession by making changes to their structure and functions by way of statutory instrument (secondary legislation) rather than by Act of Parliament (primary legislation). This allows for a quicker legislative process for changes to the function of each body. This process has been used to replace the UKCC (the former regulator for nurses and midwives) and the Council for Professions Supplementary to Medicine representing a total workforce of 750 000. The replacement bodies have smaller councils, greater lay representation, and similar functions in relation to education, conduct and registration.

This policy is supported by the influential recommendations from the Kennedy Report.[2] This commented: 'The GMC guidance on teamworking in 2000 is a sign of how much things need to change, and singularly ironic that such advice about professions working together is issued by a single professional

Table 2.1   The existing bodies that regulate health professions in the UK

Name of regulator	Professions covered	Number of regulated practitioners
Nursing and Midwifery Council	Nurses, midwives	650 000
General Medical Council	Doctors	190 000
Health Professions Council	Arts therapists, chiropodists/ podiatrists, clinical scientists, dieticians, MLSOs, occupational therapists, operating department practitioners, orthoptists, paramedics, physiotherapists, prosthetists and orthotists, radiographers, speech and language therapists	100 000
Royal Pharmaceutical Society of Great Britain	Pharmacists	40 000
General Dental Council	Dentists	34 000
General Optical Council	Opticians	18 000
General Osteopath Council	Osteopaths	2500
General Chiropractic Council	Chiropractors	1000

MLSO, medical laboratory scientific officer.

group. Multi professional teamwork needs multi professional guidance and multi professional leadership … patients do not belong to any one profession: they are the responsibility of all who take care of them.' (Ch. 22: para 45)

The concerted policy to achieve consistency in shape, function and process in the reform of the health professions regulators is appropriate for a government that is adopting an administrative role for itself in line with New Public Management. This process of reform to the individual professions will take some time and will ensure that the professions have similar approaches to education, registration and conduct. Of itself, however, it will still not be enough to consolidate the regulatory function of the state. As a result, the government's next staging post in this reform of the regulators is the creation of an overarching body that will require cooperation between the existing regulatory bodies.

The Kennedy Report supported the concept of an overarching body for the regulation of health professionals as 'an effective system of professional regulation which needs an independence from the professions and from government which allows it to act in the public interest'.[2] The new regulator, the Council for the Regulation of Health Care Professionals has been established through the NHS Reform and Regulation of Health Professions Act 2002. It will be a means to ensure consistency in approach among both existing and new healthcare professions across the UK in areas of practice, discipline and education. This overarching body will work with the current regulatory bodies to ensure that they all act in a more consistent manner. It is designed to provide for greater integration and coordination between the regulatory bodies as was made clear in the government's consultation, which said of the new body:

'It will promote continuous improvement through the setting of new performance targets and monitoring … It is clear from the Kennedy report and the experience of professional regulation in recent years that there are weaknesses in the current arrangements which need to be addressed by reforms to the individual bodies, stronger and more effective co-ordination of their work and clearer and more robust accountability mechanisms.'[33]

The government accepts that the way that the professions have been regulated is an obstacle for reform to the health service as a whole:

'The regulatory bodies will be made more accountable, open and transparent, responsive to change, with consistency of approach and greater integration and co-ordination between the regulatory bodies. The regulation of professionals needs to be flexible to facilitate new job design. The new Health Professions Council (HPC) has been established to enable extending coverage to groups of health workers not currently subject to formal statutory regulation. The redesign of jobs around the needs of patients, working across traditional professional divides, giving staff more responsibility and knowledge, focusing roles and tasks on what patients actually need in terms of their clinical care raise serious questions about the effectiveness and relevance of the present uni-professional structure of self-regulation.'[34]

REGULATION OF SETTINGS

Regulation of settings is a new approach that has been taken by the Labour government since 1997. It is further evidence of the commitment by the state to the theory of New Public Management, which requires the state to provide the framework and create executive agencies to ensure that standards can be set centrally and monitored by these agencies.

The central regulator for the NHS and arguably the most important regulator created since 1997 was the Commission for Health Improvement (CHI), which had a statutory remit to carry out inspections of every NHS facility every 4 years. The target was to carry out 500 clinical governance reviews between 2001–2004, by taking evidence from chief executives, staff and patients. Reports are published and this has led to the ability to create 'star ratings' allowing for league tables to be developed of NHS facilities. The newly created Commission for Healthcare Audit and Inspection will merge CHI with the acute private and voluntary healthcare work of the National Care Standards Commission. CHAI will also take on the value for money work of the Audit Commission, NHS complaints and the Mental Health Act Commission. Its function will be to set standards, inspect facilities and make public reports on NHS health care across England and Wales. The Commission will assess the performance of the NHS and the acute independent sector. A system of incentives will be created based on performance management so that where evidence exists that NHS facilities are treating more patients, they will earn more money from the centre. It is also evident that the use of regulatory incentives will mean that those NHS facilities that perform well will be freed from some of the more intensive regulatory regime of CHAI, particularly in the proposal to create Foundation Trusts, which will have their own regulator overseeing their establishment.

The National Care Standards Commission is the body that regulates the independent sector in both acute care and long-term care. The Registered Homes Act 1984 provided for local scrutiny and standard setting of private sector health care at health authority level. This led to wide variations on the part of the locally employed inspectors. The state-wide approach through the creation of the National Care Standards Commission set nationally required prescriptive targets that are centrally dictated and monitored by regional inspectorates throughout England. Every independent sector provider required a licence to provide healthcare services, and this is subject to annual inspection and renewal. The National Care Standards Commission sets central standards of performance that are monitored by regional inspectorates. Where a facility failed these standards, the licence could be revoked and there are provisions to revoke at short notice where it appears that patient care is dangerously unsafe. In addition, the National Care Standards Commission regulated the quality of managers that run facilities by requiring that they have achieved a certain qualification of training in management before the licence to operate in business can be effective. In this manner, the National Care Standards Commission acted as a regulator of both settings and people in a manner that is more rigorous and with greater penalties than exist for the NHS.

The principles of this national approach to regulation remain, although the regulatory structures have altered through the Health and Social Care (Community Health and Standards) Act 2003. The National Care Standards Commission is being abolished and its functions are being divided. CHAI will take on the regulation of the acute private and voluntary healthcare providers, while care homes and nursing agencies will be regulated by a new social care inspectorate, the Commission for Social Care Inspection.

The National Institute for Clinical Excellence has a remit to provide national clinical guidance. Where this guidance exists, it is likely to trump any existing guidance issued by a single regulator for a professional group.

The National Patient Safety Agency (NPSA) has a remit to develop systems that create an early warning system for the NHS. This agency was created as a result of the Chief Medical Officer's report *An Organisation with a Memory* that assessed why similar injuries that occurred to patients were not better monitored.[35] The NPSA is required to implement changes in practices that will protect patients and support staff by minimising the possibilities for human error. For instance, clearer labelling of drugs can help reduce dispensing errors and over-dosage, and tightening the procedures can minimise risk of mistakes surrounding spinal injections. There is confidentiality for staff who report incidents or near misses to the NPSA. It is not yet clear whether the level of reporting will be a matter that CHAI will take into account when it carries out its inspection of the facility. It is argued that there is a potential perverse incentive for staff to report such incidents if it is likely to have an impact on financial restriction that could be imposed by a poor CHAI report. Maintenance of confidentiality by NPSA will be a necessary means to ensure that staff have the confidence to make these reports without concern that this could impact adversely on the NHS facility.

The Health Service Commissioner for England investigates complaints against NHS trusts, primary care trusts and primary care practitioners in England, as well as investigating complaints about independent providers of health care funded by the NHS. The Health Service Commissioner accepts cases directly from complainants and has jurisdiction over the NHS with regard to maladministration and failures in providing a service, including the exercise of clinical judgement, or about the Code of Practice on Openness in the NHS. The powers and jurisdiction of the Health Service Commissioner are set out in the Health Service Commissioner Act 1993. The government is bringing together the Parliamentary Commissioner for Administration, the Health Service Commissioner and the Commission for Local Authority in England into one unified body as soon as the Parliamentary timetable allows.[36]

To implement the new regulatory regime in primary care, an independent appeal body – the Family Health Services Appeal Authority (FHSAA) – has been created to deal with appeals and applications provided for in the Health and Social Care Act 2001. The existing Family Health Services Appeal Authority (a special health authority) will continue to exist to perform adjudication functions devolved to it by the Secretary of State. The special health authority will also provide administrative services and support to the new

FHSAA. To avoid the two bodies having precisely the same name, the special health authority will in future be known as the FHSAA(SHA). Any matter on which practitioners and health authorities or primary care trusts already deal with the special health authority will continue to be dealt with by the special health authority using this new title. (Family Health Services Appeal Authority (Change of Name) Order 2001 (SI 2001/3562).

Accreditation is another form of settings regulation. Scrivens[37] traces the development of accreditation of hospitals in America in the early part of the twentieth century as a regulatory system to ensure a minimum standard of quality was reached. This system was subsequently adopted in Canada and Australia and has been adapted to include clinical performance indicators. Scrivens points out that while the initial focus of accreditation was to enable organisational development, it has increasingly become a tool of government regulation. Whether there should be accreditation of people, products (through training programmes) or settings is the issue under discussion in England. It is clear that the government has been influenced by the recommendations made in the Kennedy Report to leave less to the existing regulatory bodies that are not under the direct control of the government. For example, the Royal College of Surgeons has a duty under its Royal Charter to accredit settings where surgery is performed, but this was criticised in the Kennedy Report as being 'power without responsibility'. It is therefore likely that the government would want to ensure that it creates regulatory structures that are cohesive from the centre and which allow for a strategic approach to monitoring activity and measuring performance. If accreditation is to be used in the UK, it is likely that this will be a function of a state-created regulator working closely with employers, in both the private and NHS settings.

In England, the shift from central control and funding towards a managerial approach to health policy has meant that the government can exert central control over the creation of a regulatory framework. This provides for control of the activities of private providers of health care, as well as the creation of the performance assessment agency for the NHS. Walshe[38] maintains that these new agencies are a regulatory mechanism that allows the government to distance itself from difficult issues or unpleasant decisions without losing a hold on the work of the regulator: 'The responsibility for problems is shifted to the regulator, but the reach and scope of governmental control is retained, or even increased'. He points out that the new regulatory bodies created since 1997 share some features that confirm their role as creating the framework for performance management:

- well resourced organisations for whom regulation is the primary mission rather than one function only
- a broad remit is to oversee NHS organisations rather than a particular area
- essentially agents of the government with little independence
- all concerned primarily with clinical quality of health care rather than administrative or managerial matters.

Details of the bodies that regulate settings are shown in Table 2.2.

Table 2.2 The bodies that regulate settings

Regulator	Covers	Setting	Country
Commission for Healthcare Audit and Inspection	Service	NHS and independent acute service	England and Wales
Commission for Social Care Inspection	Service	Independent sector, nursing and care agencies	England
National Patient Safety Agency	Service	NHS	England and Wales
National Institute for Clinical Excellence	Service	NHS	England and Wales
Health Service Commissioner	Service and clinical complaints	NHS and independent sector	England
Family Health Services Appeal Authority	Doctors	NHS primary care	England

REGULATION BY EMPLOYERS

Where the state intends to implement the main framework of New Public Management, a key component is integration of employers to the policy goals. The current regulatory structure that allows the health professions regulators to determine their own standards of training and education could run counter to this strategic approach. If the government can create a direct regulatory relationship with employers, this could circumvent the need for the existing health professions regulators and ensure closer ties in the philosophy of New Public Management between state and employers in both the national and independent sectors of health care.

One clear example of the value that the government is placing on the role of the employer as regulator can be seen in the legislation that creates the new regulatory bodies for nursing and professions allied to medicine. Both regulatory bodies, the Nursing and Midwifery Council and the Health Professions Council, have a new statutory duty to cooperate with employers of healthcare professionals.

The National Clinical Assessment Authority (NCAA) is a further direct mechanism by which NHS employers can deal with underperforming doctors in acute and primary care as well as hospital dentists.[34] The NCAA is designed to complement and support the work of employers and the regulatory bodies in addressing the professional performance of individual practitioners. The Department of Health itself describes this as a 'novel approach to handling performance concerns'.[34] Rather interestingly, this novel approach was tested on hospital doctors before any other clinical group. The NCAA also provides a support forum to employers to work with them in improving the performance of individual doctors and spread good practice in the handling of competency problems. This agency's existence has been questioned:

> 'it runs the risk of being another doctor bashing instrument in what the medical profession is convinced has become a remorselessly anti doctor

environment … It will have to justify its place in the expanding spectrum of NHS performance assessment organisations. Overlap with the GMC, and the CHI is so obvious a danger that the NCAA has sought 'memoranda of understanding' with both. The proliferation of new bodies suggests inevitable rationalisation at some point and for as long as the GMC remains on probation in the minister's eyes, future changes in this area could be far reaching.'[39]

However, it appears that this agency is likely to become a place for first referral of these professions rather than the traditional route of referral to the GMC when competence is in doubt. It is possible that the role and remit of the NCAA may be the route by which the performance of doctors and dentists is managed by employers with standard setting being monitored by the state rather than the existing medical and dental regulatory bodies.

The most obvious example of the new approach being taken to shift the traditional focus of regulation of individuals can be seen in the political debate over the regulation of healthcare assistants. Healthcare assistants are not subject to any form of statutory personal regulation. The report commissioned by the government on the regulation of healthcare assistants by De Montfort University and submitted to each of the UK Departments of Health is now over 3 years old. It has still not been published. The government promised a review of regulation of healthcare assistants in the NHS Plan but has yet to produce the consultation document.[40] It can be surmised from this that the government is concerned at the implications of creating a new independent regulatory body for a large (as yet uncounted) group of individuals that will add to the myriad of bodies for individual professions in health care. New Public Management theory would suggest that employers might be best placed to police this group of workers as the most efficient mechanism for ensuring that efficiency is achieved at local level. The government recognises that employers need the flexibility to attract and monitor the workforce by a form of employer regulation that simply bypasses the traditional route of a regulatory body:

'There may be a strong case for bringing in statutory regulation for those staff whose work, increasingly unsupervised, has a direct impact on patient care. But this may be an expensive and unnecessary system to apply to all such staff. What may be needed is a range of systems, some operated by employers, specifically designed around roles and responsibilities and the training and skills needed in a patient centred NHS.'[34]

The Kennedy Report recommended that the existing Codes of Professional Conduct from the various regulatory bodies should be incorporated into the contract of employment.[2] This would allow the employer to discipline against that Code. Even though the employee who is currently regulated by a professional body will already owe various express and implied duties to the employer, which will mirror in most respects the obligations imposed on him or her by the Code of Practice, it is unclear what the rationale of this proposal is if not to give more emphasis to the role of the employer.

One of the most direct, although least publicised, mechanisms by which the government has created a direct regulatory link between state and employer is by legislation. The Protection of Children Act 1999 and the Care Standards Act 2000 create a mechanism that covers all health staff whether or not regulated by any other body. This mechanism places a statutory duty on employers to make a direct referral to the Secretary of State of staff who are considered 'unsuitable' to work with either children or vulnerable adults. Any adult receiving health care falls within the definition of vulnerable adult. This statutory duty (not a discretion) on employers is to make a referral to the Secretary of State in circumstances where there is misconduct, which harmed or placed at risk of harm a vulnerable adult or child. Where a finding is made out by the Secretary of State, that individual will be placed on a list (an 'index of unsuitable people') and prevented from working in any care setting for a period of 10 years for adults and 5 years for children. There are problems with this approach. Misconduct is not defined and could therefore involve errors not maliciously intended, such as drug errors. Where a situation technically classified as misconduct arises as a result of management failings, individuals may find themselves referred even though responsibility for failings in care should be addressed at a more systematic or a more senior level. The length of time that an individual on this Index is prevented from working in any care setting (5 years for children and 10 years for adults) provides no incentive for improvement or rehabilitation. The fixed length of sentence has no flexibility to relate to the severity of the offence. A person cleared by their own regulator from allegations of misconduct may find they are nevertheless prevented from working in a care setting by virtue of an adverse finding of misconduct by the Secretary of State.

IMPLICATIONS FOR DEVELOPMENT OF REGULATION IN ENGLAND

One advantage of the theory of New Public Management is that it accepts the political imperative that societal values and the current organisation of the health system closely prescribe which types of reform will be feasible and desirable. The extent to which the government in England has adopted the theory of New Public Management in its action and reaction to regulation of the health service is considerable since 1997. As this strategic policy is rolled out, it becomes easier to identify potential inconsistencies and overlaps that have been unconsciously designed in the regulatory structure. The construction of regulatory agencies for NHS and private healthcare settings are coherent in policy direction, are state led and directed, and are linked to dynamic and fundamental performance management across both NHS and the independent sector.

The steps taken to curtail the independence of the existing eight professional regulatory bodies has been significant and continues to move in a direction that will create more harmonisation between all professional groups, including doctors. The establishment of the overarching regulatory body to coordinate the work of the eight existing bodies has only just begun, although it is likely that its impact will be to decrease the influence of the existing professional regulatory bodies. The functions of the Council for the Regulation of Health Care Professionals will include comparing the performance of the regulatory bodies in order to promote continuous improvement by reference to each other and to other organisations. Performance improvement targets with the regulatory bodies shows that this is a form of regulation by which the state is trading individual autonomy for collective autonomy.

The role that is being given to NHS and independent sector employers by the government is significant. It would appear that this is structurally appropriate for a framework of regulation in New Public Management. Ensuring that the setting in which health care is provided is appropriately regulated requires the cooperation and alignment of employers. The steps being taken to strengthen the role of employers are consistent with this strategic approach. The advantages for the government are that it retains central control over education and standards, which will be increasingly removed from the existing regulatory bodies. Where the state creates its own standards, this in turn allows for central control of quality by ensuring that there are national methods of measuring the competencies that are achieved by clinical and non-clinical staff. In turn, those staff who demonstrate that they can improve their competencies would not be held back in a pay structure that is premised on membership of a particular professional or clinical group. The new pay structure proposed by the government for the NHS in *Agenda for Change* will allow the development of career structures that break down traditional boundaries of entry and promotion.[41]

In this revision of the regulatory arrangements, consideration should be given to how the role of the employer, strengthened by the introduction of a competency-based pay structure, will interface appropriately with any integrated regulatory system. Simply comparing performance at state level would potentially mask variations in performance across the country that could over time result in missed opportunities for continuous improvement. The scale and different sets of arrangements for the regulation of people and settings require that there is a consistent approach to performance assessment of the regulator that is not dominated by approaches designed to track the major part of the system.

The dilemma is that exaggerating external regulation may inadvertently undermine the self-confidence needed for a new social contract between government, the professions and patients. The creation of an increasingly rule-bound system is likely to inhibit risk-taking. The danger with continuing the approach developed so far is that rather than improving performance it may inadvertently undermine it. The government may create a low trust/highly regulated culture that pushes professionals into mindless compliance with protocols rather than harnessing the creativity needed to deliver high quality patient care. Rafferty[42] has argued that high trust/low-regulated organisations are more competitive. These organisations do not carry the same overheads. Quality patient experience relies upon highly committed and motivated professionals not with reference to the quality manual. The problem with the current trend is that it may squeeze out motivated and talented professionals from the NHS.

In the medium term however, it appears that the strategic policy decision to reform the health system in England along lines consistent with New Public Management has survived since 1997 and continues to form the main theoretical underpinnings of reform based on a strong central framework of regulation.

References

1 World Bank. World Bank Report. Washington, DC: World Bank; 1993.
2 Bristol Royal Infirmary Inquiry. Learning from Bristol: the report of the public inquiry into children's heart surgery at the Bristol Royal Infirmary 1984–1995 (Kennedy Report). London: The Stationery Office; 2001.
3 Secretary of State. Speech to New Health Network. London: The Stationery Office; February, 2002.
4 World Health Organization. The World Health Report 2000. Health systems: improving performance. Geneva: World Health Organization; 2000.
5 Frenk J, Donabedian A. State intervention in medical care: types, trends and variables. Health Policy Planning 1987; 2(1):17–31.
6 Robinson J. Physician–hospital integration and economic theory of the firm. Medical Care Research and Review 1997; 54(1):365–368.
7 OECD. Regulatory reform, privatisation and competition policy. OECD Report. Paris: OECD; 1992:17.
8 Williamson O. Comparative economic organisation: the analysis of discrete structural alternatives. Administrative Science Quarterly 1991; 36(June):269–296.
9 Milgrom P, Roberts J. Bargaining costs, influence costs and the organisation of economic activity. In: Alt J, Shepsle K, eds. Perspectives of positive political economy; Cambridge: Cambridge University Press; 1992:42–56.
10 Olson M. The rise and decline of nations: economic growth, stagflation and social rigidities. New Haven, CT: Yale University Press; 1982.
11 Kaul M. The new public administration: management innovations in government. Public Administration and Development 1997; 17:19–20.
12 Mackintosh M. Questioning the state. In: Wuyts M, Mackintosh M, Hewitt T, eds. Development policy and public action. Oxford: Oxford University Press; 1992:Ch. 3.
13 Mills A, Bennett S, Russell S. The challenge of health sector reform: what must governments do? Basingstoke, UK: Macmillan Press; 2001.
14 Ferlie E, Pettigrew A, Ashburner L, Fitzgerald L. The new public management in action. Oxford: Oxford University Press; 1996.
15 Girishanker N. Reforming institutions for service delivery. Policy research working paper 2039. Washington, DC: World Bank; 1999.
16 Gilson L, Mills A. Health sector reforms in sub-Saharan Africa: lessons in the last 10 years. Health Policy 1995; 32:215–243.
17 Roemer M. National health systems of the world, Vol II. Oxford: Oxford University Press; 1993.
18 Maynard A. The regulation of public and private health care markets. In: McLachlan G, Maynard A, eds. A public/private mix for health: the relevance and effects of change. London: Nuffield Provincial Hospitals Trust; 1982:28–45.
19 Posner R. Theories of economic regulation. Bell Journal of Economics and Management Science 1974; 5(2):335–358.
20 Selznick P. Focusing organisational research on regulation. In: Noll R, ed. Regulatory policy and the social sciences. Berkeley: University of California Press; 1985:363–368.

21 Kumaranayake L. The role of regulation: influencing private sector activity within health reform. Journal of International Development 1997; 9(4):641–649.

22 Bennett S, Dakpallah G, Garner P, et al. Carrot and stick: state mechanisms to influence private provider behaviour. Health Policy and Planning 1994; 9(1):1–13.

23 Stiglitz J. The economic role of the state. Oxford: Basil Blackwell; 1989.

24 Bennett S. The mystique of markets: public and private health care in developing countries. PHP Departmental Publication No. 4. London: London School of Hygiene and Tropical Medicine; 1991.

25 Kumaranayake L. Economic aspects of health sector regulation: strategic choices for low and middle income countries. PHP Departmental Publication No. 29. London: London School of Hygiene and Tropical Medicine; 1998.

26 Norton E. Incentive regulation of nursing homes. Journal of Health Economics 1992; 11:105–128.

27 Secretary of State. Speech to NHS Confederation Conference. Harrogate: Secretary of State; 2002:May.

28 Davies C. What about the girl next door? Gender and the politics of professional self regulation. In: Bendelow G et al., eds. Gender health and healing. London: Routledge; 2001:69–85.

29 Friedson E. Profession of medicine: a study of the sociology of applied knowledge. New York: Dodd, Mead; 1970.

30 National Consumer Council. Self regulation of professionals in health care. London: National Consumer Council; 1999.

31 Consumers Association. Professional self-regulation; a patient centred approach. Consultation document. London: Consumers Association; 2000.

32 Pyne R. Professional regulation: shaken but not stirred. Consumer Policy Review 2000; 10(5):167–173.

33 Department of Health. Modernising regulation in the health professions. Consultation. London: Department of Health; 2001:August.

34 Department of Health. HR strategy for England. Consultation. London: Department of Health; 2002:April–July.

35 Department of Health. An organisation with a memory. Report of an expert group on learning from adverse events in the NHS. London: The Stationery Office; 2000.

36 Health Services Commission. Job advert for health services commissioner. Law Society Gazette 2002; April.

37 Scrivens E. International trends in accreditation. Journal of Health Planning and Management 1995; 10:165–181.

38 Walshe K. The rise of regulation in the NHS. British Medical Journal 2002; 324:967–970.

39 Editorial. Health Services Journal 2001; 15 November:17.

40 Department of Health. NHS plan for England. London: The Stationery Office; 2000.

41 Department of Health. Agenda for change, the new NHS pay system – an overview, London: Department of Health; 2003.

42 Rafferty A-M. Risk and trust in the NHS: Modernising regulation – can we still trust health professionals? Address to Kings Fund, 2001.

Chapter 3

Cost implications and ethics of healthcare quality regulation

Stephen Heasell

INTRODUCTION

This chapter is about how cost implications of healthcare quality regulation might affect its outcomes. The discussion is illustrated with reference mainly to the case of the National Health Service (NHS) in the UK. Reference is made particularly to the English law of clinical negligence and to the development of clinical guidelines within a broader vision of NHS governance.

This chapter identifies ways in which various costs are, or could be, taken into account in devising, implementing and responding to aspects of healthcare quality regulation. It offers an explanation, grounded in the economic principle of social scarcity among valuable resources, of why the scope for maintaining or improving the quality of health care will usually be determined partly by cost and hence why there is always a case in favour of considering quality and cost together for policy purposes.

The chapter also suggests that controversy about evaluating quality, cost and cost effective quality in health care will persist, largely because different ethical or other perspectives are brought to bear by various interested parties on how it should be done and where the costs should fall.

The reformed NHS governance and the law of clinical negligence have been chosen as two contrasting, but potentially linked types of regulation to investigate the following propositions:

- Regulation of healthcare *quality* is also about healthcare *costs*.
- Every interested party takes *cost effectiveness* into account in some way when devising, implementing or responding to healthcare quality regulation.
- The scope for maintaining or improving the quality of health care in the UK by regulation depends on stimulating the cost effective use of the resources available to the NHS.
- The pursuit of cost effectiveness in the context of the NHS raises ethical and other concerns and there remains no social consensus about how to pursue it.
- Particular prescriptions of a socially responsible way to measure cost effectiveness in the context of healthcare regulation cannot be expected to command an effective social consensus.

REGULATION, QUALITY AND COST: THE NHS CONTEXT

The Wanless Report about long-term requirements for the NHS[1] was issued on 17 April 2002, the same day as the annual Budget Report speech for 2002 by the Chancellor of the Exchequer.[2] Together, these two presentations clearly constituted a challenge to the NHS to demonstrate its cost effectiveness.

Considerable increases in the overall NHS budgets planned for several years ahead were announced, coupled with expectations that the broad objective of a more consistently satisfactory overall quality of service will be demonstrated. Many differences of opinion may well be expressed or harboured quietly about what constitutes or counts as a more consistently satisfactory quality of service. Some of these opinions will be principled, others pragmatic. A clear link, nevertheless, was being made by the Chancellor and in Wanless between the wherewithal to pay for extra real resources for the NHS (hence the costs of it) and some demonstrable evidence of extra effectiveness, however effectiveness is to be interpreted and however the demonstration is to be made.

This stance appears to recognise that versatile resources remain scarce and that money is not the only scarce resource. Indeed, the recent record of NHS budgets remaining unspent by the end of the relevant accounting period suggests that, in the short term, some employable labour skills and elements of infrastructure may be scarcer than the money with which to pay for them.

There seems to be some agreement that, if the UK is to rely on the NHS to deliver the healthcare quality to which it aspires, considerable increases in the NHS budget will be required. In other words, the NHS will cost considerably more than the nation has been spending on it and more as a proportion of national income. This would imply that a correspondingly lower proportion of national income and possibly a lower budget in real terms would be devoted to other things. A connection therefore has been made between increased cost and enhanced fulfilment of aspirations (that is, between cost and effectiveness in some broad sense).

It also seems to be agreed, however, at least by the Chancellor of the Exchequer and in the Wanless Report, that a considerable increase in the budget alone will not guarantee effectiveness in the form of fulfilling those aspirations. The Wanless Report indicates explicitly that the size of NHS budget required will depend on how the budget is spent. The Chancellor anticipated that the internal NHS processes which influence its spending patterns will change, and will have to change, if the increased budget is to bring demonstrable improvements in overall healthcare quality. If the increased funding is sustained but demonstrable improvements are not forthcoming, then it will become more difficult to rally support for basing the delivery of health services on a set of institutions that draw on the traditions of the NHS.

The existence of healthcare quality *regulation*, in various forms as it affects individuals and organisations, suggests that regulators (at least) believe hope and individual self-determination alone to be insufficient for delivering sufficient impact. Regulation implies that particular responsibilities are allocated to particular people or organisations and that they are then held accountable for upholding those responsibilities. Regulation may be presented as a way to promote healthcare quality but, given the connections made explicitly between increased cost and increased fulfilment of aspirations for the NHS, that implies attention to cost effectiveness (in some sense) for the pursuit of healthcare quality in the way regulation is designed and imposed.

It is of course possible to question whether these points of apparent agreement are logically inescapable, if not also to reconsider them on empirical, ethical or other grounds. For example, if a healthcare organisation is sufficiently wasteful of its opportunities, there could be scope henceforth to improve quality and also to reduce total costs.

COST EFFECTIVENESS: AN INDIVIDUAL'S PERSPECTIVE

If the notion of cost effectiveness is to be taken successfully into account for purposes of healthcare policy, then its interpretation as above at the level of the nation as a whole will be linked with its interpretation for individual decision making. Individuals routinely consider whether or not deployment of their time, energies and attributes (or money) to some thing or some activity in particular would be worthwhile. Each of them can thus be said to use a cost effectiveness criterion in their decision making about the NHS or health care as about other matters. Ultimately, the decision may vary according to whether or not the individual expects to reap all the benefits of the thing or activity in question, or incur all the costs, but arguably the criterion of cost effectiveness remains. Both costs and effectiveness might be considered purely in terms of material inputs and outcomes or could include intangible ones. The intangibles could include the merits or otherwise of the process by which outcomes are generated as distinct from those of the outcomes themselves. They could also include compliance with ethical criteria, which might embrace notions of equity, the fulfilment of a duty or the exercise of an opportunity. If so, then costs and effectiveness become increasingly difficult to measure precisely and explicitly but arguably they are still being considered together, somehow, in making a decision. Indeed, a decision not to refine a cost effectiveness calculation any further, on the grounds that the extra effort would not be worthwhile, could be said in itself to be a practical application of the criterion. If so, rhetorical objections on ethical grounds to the use of a cost effectiveness criterion in the NHS require careful consideration.

Even if it is the case that every individual routinely uses a cost effectiveness yardstick in their own decision making about health care, however, that would not necessarily prevent objections by the individual, principled or pragmatic, to attempts by others to impose a particular version of that yardstick. We can expect every individual, from their various personal perspectives, to evaluate elements of cost and effectiveness differently. Indeed, it is likely that individuals employ a much more versatile and flexible conception of costs in conducting their own cost effectiveness analysis for themselves than is found in any standard index compiled for public purposes. Criticisms of using the criterion in regulating NHS practice may, therefore, miss the mark. Instead, it may simply be a shorthand way of objecting to a particular version of the criterion, or to the way it is implemented or to the consequences of its implementation for some people.

The pursuit of cost effectiveness then could be an attempt by individuals to achieve the cost effective way to satisfy ethical or other considerations in using the limited resources at their command. The ethical perspectives adopted might include perceptions of what constitutes justice in the distribution of wealth, welfare or opportunity between people, presumably including the individual currently in command of the resources. In this sense, distributional justice can be pursued effectively and efficiently or otherwise. Cost effectiveness and efficiency can be interpreted in terms of a moral or ethical imperative, if to be inefficient is unnecessarily to waste opportunities to achieve distributional justice.

Objections by an individual to a version of cost effectiveness adopted by others are all the more likely to occur if that version seems obscure and difficult or time consuming to understand, either in principle or in the detail of practical application. Arguably, economists have done more than most to make principled analysis seem more obscure than necessary. Sometimes this occurs in the attempt to take a number of individual perspectives all into account simultaneously in one concise indicator of cost effectiveness. The development in recent years of health indices such as the quality adjusted life year (known as the QALY), hence estimates of cost per QALY (health) gained from healthcare interventions, is just one prominent case in point. Any concise single indicator conceals many of the controversies inherent both among those various perspectives and in the process of combining them.

There is certainly a risk that a focus on demonstrable cost effectiveness would reduce the decision making process to one that is geared exclusively to a very unsubtle version of an economic efficiency objective and one which overrides a plurality of criteria that might embrace alternative notions of equity and justice. This risk is increased if quick and explicit decision making is required because the indicators of cost effectiveness that will be available most readily and at least cost will include the least subtle ones. An unsophisticated adoption of these unsubtle indicators could even be defended, with some superficial plausibility, by claiming that anything more ambitious would almost certainly cost more but might not in practice yield any extra benefits.

For the time being at least the government has explicitly embraced both the use of the cost effectiveness criterion in NHS governance and also the inclusion of research-based evidence in using that criterion. Rhetorical objections to this will receive short shrift. If the criterion is interpreted strictly claims, or even research-based evidence, that a particular NHS practice is effective for one or more patients will not be accepted as sufficient to show that any of the NHS budget should be spent on it. Any such claims or objections would instead be judged according to whether or not there is good reason to believe that they point the way to improving the effectiveness of the NHS, public spending or health care, as a whole.

REGULATION OF QUALITY BY LAW, GOVERNANCE AND GUIDELINES

Elements in the regulation of healthcare quality are presented by their champions as ways to maintain and improve quality. This applies to contrasting forms of regulation, including the vision of NHS governance that has been promoted by Labour governments since 1997.[3] It also applies to the law of clinical negligence, to which considerable numbers of NHS patients turn hoping, it is often said, among other things to prevent injuries in the future to others.

Some other elements in regulation are presented, by their champions or their opponents, as ways to contain spending on health care. Some of the many sets of clinical guidelines in the United States for example have been seen as agents of cost containment[4] and the terms of reference for the National Institute for Clinical Excellence (NICE) in the UK, when appraising clinical products or services for the purpose of generating authoritative clinical guidelines, make mention of cost-effectiveness criteria as well as clinical-effectiveness criteria.[3] Commentators have observed that, whether considerations of quality or cost are uppermost, effective regulation of governance imposes some form of healthcare rationing. This is because it affects the allocation of limited budgets to health care and between different uses in health care.[5]

A common denominator between these different elements of healthcare quality regulation is that both quality enhancement and cost containment are pursued typically by seeking a way to allocate responsibility between various parties for achieving these purposes and holding the responsible parties to account for doing so. This approach is found in regulation of various forms as well as regulation for various purposes.

In allocating these responsibilities, quality regulation inevitably also allocates between the parties a burden of costs, or the risk of incurring particular costs, in one guise or another. Those held responsible for promoting healthcare quality incur costs either if they strive to improve quality or if they strive merely to appear to do so or if they are held to account for not doing so. The responses of those to be held accountable will also influence the costs (or risks of costs) incurred by other parties including patients depending on how the health care actually made available is affected by regulation.

If a particular allocation of responsibilities for healthcare quality does affect the allocation of costs in some way, then it becomes relevant to ask a series of questions about whether or how this connection influences the achievement of regulatory purposes. These questions include whether or how regulators take costs explicitly into account when they allocate responsibilities for healthcare quality. Issues about whether or how they *should* do so also become relevant.

In the highly politicised context of NHS health care, central government has a continuing interest in demonstrating convincingly that the limited but expanding NHS budget delivers an increasingly satisfactory service. Such a demonstration remains difficult to achieve while an impression remains among the electorate that NHS care varies widely in quality, including some which is unnecessarily ineffective or worse. That impression is likely to persist if claims and awards in respect of clinical negligence remain so prominently in the media spotlight.[6]

The NHS budget, limited as it is by rival claims for government spending and by perceptions of a limited public tolerance of taxation, makes cost effectiveness in using the budget an essential determinant of the scope for delivering overall levels of public service including health care of an acceptable quality. A failure to be cost effective within a budget of any size would limit the opportunities to deliver an increasingly satisfactory service, if levels of satisfaction are correlated positively with levels of service. It cannot be surprising then if regulation of healthcare quality that is instigated by UK governments is done in a way which seeks to promote cost effective health care as well as examples of high quality health care.

NHS GOVERNANCE AND TORT LAW

The NHS governance framework now emerging and the tort law of clinical negligence are two distinctive forms of regulation of healthcare activity, both of which address the issue of unsatisfactory quality. They are ultimately alternative forms of regulation (substitutes for each other at least partially and at the margin), with different regulators sitting in judgement, but they might also be complementary with each other. They could mutually reinforce a set of incentives to contain the costs of negligence. In particular, NHS activity remains subject to claims under tort law and as a result NHS governance is designed so as to influence the actions of clinicians and others such that these claims are moderated. Both governance and the tort law, together or individually, affect the allocation of resources between different uses in health care, including the allocation of risk, rights and responsibilities. In doing so, they also affect the distribution of resources and hence wealth between people, together with their welfare and opportunities. At issue is the extent to which these effects on allocation or distribution reflect the purposes set for the two types of regulation by design or are merely incidental side effects of pursuing other purposes.

INTEGRATION, INFORMATION AND INCENTIVES WITHIN NHS GOVERNANCE

The Wanless Report[1] contains suggestions, based on a review of NHS practice, about what will affect the size of the budgets required if broad objectives for the service are to be met. Themes of integration, information and incentives loom large among these suggestions. The implication is that if more attention is not paid to these themes than hitherto then the budget cost of future NHS overall effectiveness will be that much higher. A further implication is that it would be worthwhile to spend some of the increased budgets on ways to improve integration, information and incentives even though to do so would initially divert those resources from the products and activities at the frontline of healthcare delivery. Such a balance of priorities would appear to endorse attempts to reform NHS governance by improving, in particular, the evidence base together with its dissemination within and across the NHS. It also seems to endorse, however, the provision of improved incentives to take responsibility for upholding the quality of NHS care. The incentives could take the form of welcome and positive carrots or else negative big sticks. Sceptics might ask whether Wanless and the advocates of investments in NHS governance have subjected their own prescriptions to the test of cost effectiveness as rigorously as they advocate should be done for other NHS spending proposals.

The apparatus of governance now being developed and established at the instigation of the Labour government amounts to a reformed regulatory regime for the NHS. It seems to reflect a view that, for one reason or another, individuals respond to incentives inherent in the way the employment of their services is organised so that systematic attention to the incentives generated by that organisation is essential if any particular social objective is to be achieved.

Even if there were to be a broad consensual commitment to ensure best overall use of resources, taking many possible uses and users into account in the allocation process, then individual and localised perceptions alone would not necessarily achieve it. This problem could be construed charitably as one of limited local information and divergent interests, leading to imperfect overall coordination of activity. Under some conditions, competition for resources by market exchange between individuals (competitive market forces) might serve to establish the relevant coordination. If that possibility is rejected, an alternative is to try to do so by means of planning and regulation of some kind, which includes a degree of centralised authority. NHS governance, by that or any other name, has always combined a considerable element of centralised authority with some individual and local discretion in various degrees. By contrast, an upsurge of attempts to stimulate competition in markets for NHS resources occurred in the 1980s and 1990s although in a way that also involved considerable centralised regulation to sustain it.

The components of NHS governance currently include National Service Frameworks (NSF) and quality assurance obligations for the organisations that comprise the NHS as a whole, together with the Commission for Health Improvement (CHI) and the NICE. They also include a set of guidelines, some of them drawn up or kite marked by the NICE. They are to be joined by the Commission for Healthcare Audit and Inspection (CHAI). These components can be interpreted as contributions in various ways and degrees to the information and incentive elements of governance. The main terms of reference set out for the NICE involve the summary and dissemination of information about cost effectiveness of clinical practice based on research evidence. This information is to be incorporated into clinical guidelines which, along with financial and other guidelines, fit within those of the NSF. Together, they begin to offer a basis for both an appraisal of NHS prospects and for the audit of NHS performance in terms of cost effectiveness. This agenda for the NICE represents a monumental task if it is to be done fully and well. To date, only patchy research evidence is available about many aspects of NHS care and NHS performance indicators by and large have hitherto not been related closely to cost-effective fundamental outcomes.

Incentives for NHS governance, hence cost-effective quality in the NHS, are provided partly by the CHI with its various powers of investigation and intervention. These powers include ultimately the replacement of local managers and management. Incentives are also inherent in the basis on which the overall NHS budget is allocated to various uses and users, including the ways in which local organisations are paid for their services. Payment methods will increasingly be designed to reward effective performance among those given some discretion to decide how to be effective. Payments are less likely to be made exclusively for nominal activities undertaken or for expenditures incurred.

The theme of integration, particularly amongst providers of health and related social services, poses particular challenges for the provision of both information and incentives. Common access to the same comprehensive body of evidence-based information might be an advantage but the evidence would then have to be all the more extensive and complex to cover all cases and using it in decision making would be made that much more difficult.

Integration is less likely to occur if the organisational incentives facing the various interested parties are misaligned. The incentives may appear to be perverse when viewed in terms of objectives that go beyond one particular component organisation. Piecemeal changes in arrangements within a large and complicated organisation like the NHS can have unforeseen incentive effects in and beyond the part targeted for change, largely because changes in resource allocation take place that have wider implications.

There may be some advantages in adopting a broader perspective by devising changes in organisational arrangements from Olympian heights at or beyond the centre of the NHS. Their effectiveness would be undermined, however, unless an adequate understanding exists at the centre about how the arrangements affect incentives locally and unless there is a systematic approach to setting those incentives.

A recurrent feature of the debate about the future of the NHS has concerned its responsiveness to patients. An argument for expanding the role of patient choice, even if not by patients acting fully as paying consumers in a market for NHS care, is that it would provide a flow of decentralised information and incentives to NHS providers that did not rely quite so heavily for its success on the NHS at the centre (or the government) to make sense of all the detail.

In the NHS, the job of balancing the preferences of individual current patients with the interests of all taxpayers, who between them ultimately fund most of the service, will remain a centralised responsibility, while clinical decision making will remain substantially the devolved responsibility of clinicians even if legal liability is shared with others. The promotion of increased patient choice highlights a tension that was designed into the NHS from its inception, between the interests of individual patients and the more collective aspects of healthcare provision in the UK. Only within a well-designed NHS governance as a whole could the information and incentives flowing from expanded individual choice cut the costs of resolving that tension.

COST EFFECTIVENESS AND THE LAW OF CLINICAL NEGLIGENCE

The tort law of clinical negligence has the effect of imposing costs on interested parties in various ways, most obviously when court awards are made and when lawyers are paid. Less obviously, it has also been suggested[7] that court judgments made according to the tort law on negligence have the effect of promoting cost effectiveness in the provision of health care. This suggestion has been made most prominently about the legal (and health care) context of the USA, following the work of Posner,[8,9] but has also been made in the English context.[10] In both cases, doubt is cast on whether court judgments consistently reflect any particular redistributive purpose, equitable or otherwise, and on whether the tort law would be the most efficient vehicle for doing so compared with the alternatives. It can also be noted that tort law, evolving as it does over the long term from case to case, may not be a consistent reflection of any particular policy of any particular government.

The criterion of cost effectiveness in the context of clinical negligence can be presented as an attempt to minimise the sum of the costs that could arise from two sources: from the occurrence of clinical error (or patient injury more generally) and from attempts to avoid such an error (or injury). It can be envisaged that a balance between these two sets of costs will be considered by various interested parties, in their own way, among them the providers of clinical services. If the costs of injury and the costs of avoidance both rise at increasing rates the more that injury or attempts to avoid injury occur, then it is predictable that the sum of these costs will be minimised as soon as an extra pound spent on avoiding injury would save less than a pound on the costs of injury.[11] If court judgments reflected this criterion of cost effectiveness, then judgments would be made in favour of the patient if the provider of services had not done enough to minimise the sum of those costs. If these court judgments served the cause of cost-effective quality of health care, then they would do so by acting as an incentive to providers in the future to minimise the relevant sum of costs. The judgments would act as a cost effective deterrent to clinical injury by drawing forth cost effective levels of precaution against injury, not maximum possible precautions. If the rate of judgments made in favour of patients increased, or if the size of court awards to patients increased, other things being equal, then providers of services would deploy more of their resources in spending to avoid injury. In addition, or instead, they might seek to settle more claims by offering a sum in compensation before a court judgment is made and hence hope to avoid some legal costs.

In 2002, The National Audit Office (NAO) reported an increase of about half a billion pounds sterling in one year in the NHS provisions for costs arising from clinical negligence claims.[6] The NHS Litigation Authority has emerged in recent years as a prominent influence on clinical risk management processes in the NHS. The reformed NHS governance includes the allocation of other relevant responsibilities for quality assurance, among them an assiduous reporting of adverse events. Each of these developments could be consistent with the achievement of cost effective health care, if any additional costs incurred in seeking to avoid negligence or claims of negligence are more than outweighed, either by cost reductions as fewer cases and claims arise or by better outcomes of the health care provided. The NAO noted that the rate of increase of NHS provisions, while still giving rise to concern, had slowed down compared with previous years.

Posner, who in the USA has occupied the posts of Supreme Court Judge and Professor of Economics simultaneously, suggests that the law of negligence does indeed serve the cause of cost effectiveness or at least one version of it. If all the negative features of the risk of medical injury can be aggregated and represented as a cost by a money sum (perhaps to identify appropriate compensation to the injured parties) and if every pound's worth of cost is regarded as being equivalent in value, then a comparison between costs of injury and costs of injury avoidance could be made. This would enable a judgement to be reached about whether or not a provider of care had striven sufficiently to uphold a quality of service that would minimise the sum of these costs. Reference has been made, for example, to the use in US courts from 1947 of the so-called Hand Formula.[12] By that formula, the reasonableness or otherwise of care provided would be considered according to whether the cost of avoidance exceeded the value of harm caused by any injury, weighted by its probability of occurrence. The plausibility of explaining court judgments as being an attempt to achieve cost effective outcomes turns on a number of issues. It depends, first, on what is included as a cost and how the costs are combined into a single sum. The acceptability of including only those costs where money actually changes hands and of counting each pound of costs equally, which might serve in those cases where promotion of money wealth in business is a key concern, seems especially weak in some cases involving major injury to health.

The plausibility of the Posner explanation also depends on how well informed the courts are. For example, the more that regulators rely on the individuals or the organisations that are being regulated as a source of information, the more vulnerable are those regulators to seeing the circumstances of the case from the particular perspective of those who are regulated and their judgement being affected accordingly. This phenomenon is known as regulatory capture and care would be needed to avoid it if, for example, sources of relevant clinical expertise were limited to a particularly close-knit group of practitioners. NHS clinicians and managers of necessity have some privileged access to some relevant information by virtue of their technical expertise and in their role as agent both for individual patients and also for the NHS as an organisation.

Existence of authoritative clinical guidelines as a component of NHS governance, based on research evidence of best practice from various sources including those beyond the NHS, could reduce the impact of regulatory capture although the guidelines are NHS guidelines and the NICE is an NHS body. Arguably, therefore, these arrangements constitute a type of internal self-regulation without a wholly independent element to it and hence tantamount to regulatory capture. There are some signs that guidelines are having an influence on court cases,[13] although the firm evidence to date seems limited if not uncertain. Guidelines within NHS governance are not mandatory and they do not remove responsibility from clinicians for clinical judgement in individual cases.

Another issue, arguably linked to that of regulatory capture, is the standard of care. Under English law, providers of clinical services are held by the courts to a standard of practice according to the so-called Bolam Test (*Bolam* v. *Friern Hospital Management Committee* [1957] 1 WLR 583) and now also in the light of the Bolitho case (*Bolitho* v. *City and Hackney HA* [1988] AC 232). The relevant standard of care is one whereby a practitioner would not be considered negligent by a responsible body of medical opinion, even if there is another responsible body of opinion that would take a different view. Bolitho indicates that there are circumstances where a judge can conclude that a practice is not responsible, notwithstanding that it has been endorsed by an expert witness in the relevant specialty, because it does not stand up to logical scrutiny.[13] This may or may not imply, however, that the standard of practice required reflects a criterion that takes into account costs other than those perceived by clinicians. The admissibility of more than one medical body of opinion suggests that should cost effectiveness be used as a criterion at all there is no consensus on which version of it to use even among clinicians.

The explanation of the law of clinical negligence as a type of regulation that facilitates cost effective quality of health care remains controversial and questionable, even in the US context. It is all the more questionable in the peculiar British context of the NHS, where the free flow of market forces for the allocation of resources for most health care has explicitly been rejected. It does, nevertheless, help to show that a variety of ways to decide on what quality of health care to uphold could each be constructed or construed as a version of the cost effectiveness criterion. That is not to say, in a world of rival claims for scarce resources, that any single version of the criterion would command an enthusiastic or effective consensus.

CONCLUSION

It does not seem credible that the narrowest standardised interpretation of the cost effectiveness criterion will completely dominate decision making in health care. There are too many alternative versions of that criterion, and possibly other criteria, being acted upon by too many people, some of them powerful ones, for that to happen.

It could well be, nevertheless, that a restricted version of cost effectiveness will hold increased sway in decision making. That might be because of the influence of various regulators, including governments and the courts. It could also be because it is becoming technically easier than before to implement an evidence-based indicator with costs measured in standard ways in money terms. Hitherto, interested parties could claim, perhaps with some plausibility, that such a standardised approach to decision making was impractical whatever its other attractions.

References

1 Wanless D. Securing our future health: taking a long-term view. Final report. London: HM Treasury; 2002.
2 HM Treasury Budget Report. London; 2002: April. Online. Available: http://www.treasury.gov.uk/Budget/bud_bud02/bud_bud02_index.cfm
3 Heasell SL. The economics of clinical guidelines. In: Tingle J, Foster C, eds. Clinical guidelines: law, policy and practice. London: Cavendish; 2002:181–198.
4 Solomon RP. Clinical guidelines in the United States: perspectives on law and litigation. In: Tingle J, Foster C, eds. Clinical guidelines: law, policy and practice. London: Cavendish; 2002:137–160.
5 Norheim OF. Clinical guidelines: healthcare rationing and accountability for reasonableness. In: Tingle J, Foster C, eds. Clinical guidelines: law, policy and practice. London: Cavendish; 2002:161–180.
6 National Audit Office. NHS (England) Summarised accounts 2000–2001, HC 766 2001–2002; 2002.
7 Danzon P. Medical malpractice: theory, practice and public policy. Cambridge, Massachusetts: Harvard University Press; 1985.
8 Posner R. Economic analysis of law. Boston: Little Brown; 1992.
9 Posner R. Theory of negligence. Journal of Legal Studies 1982; 1:29–96.
10 Towse A, Danzon P. Medical negligence and the NHS: an economic analysis. Health Economics 1999; 8:93–101.
11 Calabresi G. The costs of accidents: a legal and economic analysis. New Haven: Yale University Press; 1970.
12 Dnes AW. The economics of law. London: International Thomson Business; 1996:126–127.
13 Tingle J. The developing role of clinical guidelines. In: Tingle J, Foster C, eds. Clinical guidelines: law, policy and practice. London: Cavendish; 2002:99–111.

Chapter 4

Fault and blame in the NHS: review and replacement of the clinical negligence system in the UK

Timothy James

'Clinical negligence is not a good system. But the alternatives may not achieve the benefits claimed for them and there is an ethical price to be paid, which many of their enthusiasts do not seem to have considered.'

INTRODUCTION

A number of mechanisms, internal and external, are intended to secure the delivery of high quality health care in England and Wales. Internally, there are protocols, management structures, clinical audit and the like. Externally, mechanisms include professional registration for the various health professions and inspection by bodies such as the Commission for Health Improvement (CHI) and the National Patient Safety Agency (NPSA); but perhaps the most controversial quality mechanism external to the service is the law of clinical negligence.

Of course, the clinical negligence system is much more than a healthcare quality mechanism; but one of the policy reasons for which we apply the same principles of skill and care to health professionals as to others is that it is believed that the prospect of personal liability to compensate the injured will encourage error prevention. This, it is hoped, will raise quality.

Negligence is part of the law of tort and the fundamental concept behind the tort of negligence is breach of a duty to take care. Lawyers technically refer to breach of duty as 'fault'. No doubt we require those 'at fault' to compensate those injured by their failure to take care because of a sense of moral responsibility; but it is also felt to be good policy, because it encourages people to be careful for their own sake and it takes the burden of compensation off those who were not at fault.

THE HISTORY OF REFORM

Against a background of near panic at the increasing number and value of claims for clinical negligence, there have been numerous calls for radical reform, even abolition, of the fault-based system of compensation for medical mishaps. These calls have, in recent times, generally been coupled with arguments that the culture of health care is too preoccupied with blame and that a blame-free culture would actually tend to provide a higher quality of care. These arguments have been urged by many parties, but most frequently by or on behalf of medical practitioners and other clinicians.[1]

Such calls were initially resisted by UK governments: as recently as 1998 the then Health Minister, Paul Boateng, clearly and apparently decisively rejected no-fault compensation in Parliament.[2] But, by late 2001, persistence had succeeded in moving the government at least to consider abolition as a serious option. The breakthrough for the pro-abolitionists was, almost certainly, the recommendation of abolition by Professor (now Sir) Ian Kennedy in his report into the Bristol paediatric heart surgery scandal.[3] This combined a high-profile and intensely emotive issue with a thorough and powerful argument for its recommendation. Professor Kennedy did not, however, recommend in detail what should replace fault.

A consultation was set up, with the stated object of making the system faster and fairer, for patients and healthcare professionals. Professor Liam Donaldson, the Chief Medical Officer for England, chaired it and the membership was made up of six healthcare professionals and managers, six lawyers and civil servants and three patients' representatives. It was also intended to reform the NHS complaints procedure, promote rapid non-financial remedies, increase learning from mistakes and reduce the cost of negligence claims. Specific questions upon which consultation was sought included: which no-fault schemes should be examined; whether there should be fixed tariffs for specific injuries; whether the negligence and complaints systems could be integrated; whether claims could be limited to the cost of NHS, rather than private care; whether indemnities, rather than lump sum damages, could be given; and how to change the funding of how claims are made, to control costs.

The consultation commenced in October 2001.[4] A White Paper was promised early in 2002, but it was not until June 2003 that Professor Donaldson issued a report entitled *Making Amends*, described as a consultation paper with proposals for reform.[5] It did not recommend abolition, but proposed a system to lie alongside clinical negligence which was explicitly intended drastically to reduce the incidence of litigation.[6] It is the purpose of this chapter to examine some of the implications of the Kennedy/Donaldson proposals; it is not intended to be a detailed analysis of *Making Amends*.

A note on terminology

A number of terms are closely associated in discussing this issue and before proceeding we need to note their overlaps and their differences. In particular, we must note that the legal concept of *fault* and the more general phenomenon of *blame*, are linked but not identical.

When a word in general usage becomes a term of art for a professional, the lay listener is prone to misunderstand it. When a lawyer says someone is 'at fault', a non-lawyer may well see this as exactly the same as saying that that person is personally to blame for what went wrong. The non-lawyer may object to this on the ground that many other factors were involved in causing the error. Because we generally blame those who are at fault, we tend to use the terms interchangeably.

But this is to miss the point of the lawyer's statement, which may well be a technical one, not intended to carry any moral blame. For example, a doctor exhausted by too many nights on call who miswrites a drug dosage is subject in the law's eyes to exactly the same standard of care as a fully-rested colleague and so is 'at fault' (in the lawyer's sense), even if we can hardly blame the doctor, rather than the system, for the error. Conversely, we may rightly blame a doctor who is rude and patronising, but this would not normally be a fault in the lawyer's sense.

To illustrate the distinction, try to imagine a no-blame system and a no-fault system, and reflect on the difference.

In a *no-blame* system, errors would no doubt occur and sometimes they would be someone's fault, but we would avoid attributing moral responsibility to individuals, in order to encourage full and frank reporting of and learning from the error.

In a *no-fault* system, the same number of errors would presumably occur and individuals might be considered morally responsible, but this would be irrelevant to the question of compensation, which would depend on other issues, such as the avoidability of the error and the amount of harm caused.

Blame, in other words, is a general psychological reaction of all of us and we can at best take a self-denying resolve to resist it, or at least not to act on it inappropriately; but fault is a legal or ethical attribution of personal responsibility, the legal and other consequences of which we can build into our compensation system or not as we choose, on policy grounds.

A *no-error* system is universally recognised to be an impossible dream.

JUSTIFICATIONS FOR REFORM

The justifications offered for replacing our current fault-based compensation system include:

- the financial burden on healthcare providers of paying compensation reduces the resources available for health care (the total cost of meeting current claims as at the end of March 2002 was estimated by the National Audit Office (NAO) at £5.25 billion[7])[i]

- artificial difficulties are placed in the way of the claims of some deserving parties by legal technicalities – for example, the outcomes of factually indistinguishable cases can depend on the different skill levels of the expert witnesses called. It is estimated by the NAO that only 24% of legally aided claims are successful[8]
- fear of liability tends to cause healthcare professionals to practice 'defensive medicine'[9,10]
- a fault-based system places disproportionate emphasis on errors by individuals, when the true causes of injury are complex systemic factors in healthcare organisations[11–13]
- though good at achieving some of the range of objectives of claimants, such as financial compensation and, arguably, punishment, they are poor at others, such as obtaining admissions of wrongdoing and improvement of the system for future users (the NHS complaints procedure, for example, positively bars those pursuing financial compensation from simultaneously seeking an explanation, apology or assurances as to the future)
- they are relatively inefficient for the solution of small and medium sized claims. It is frequently noted that in claims under £50 000, the costs of settlement often exceed the damages awarded.[8]

To these might be added the following criticisms of fault-based systems, which have in practice been less canvassed:

- they rely on memory or record-keeping, both of which are prone to incompleteness and to retrospective distortion
- they are even worse at achieving other desirable ends, such as the clearing of the innocent – 'mud sticks'
- most damning, the persistence of serious medical error, despite numerous initiatives to reduce or eliminate it (the NAO cites evidence that estimates rates of preventable adverse events at 5% of all acute hospital admissions[14]), shows that pressurizing individuals by the fear of liability is, in practice, ineffective in increasing the quality of health care delivered and may indeed actually be counter-productive.

The main arguments

However, the most cogent arguments for abolition or radical reform have claimed at least one (usually both) of the following benefits for a system based on a principle other than fault:

1 the acquisition of fuller and more timely information about the causation of adverse events, which will make it possible to reduce the future incidence of such events; and

---

[i]The amount actually paid out during 2001–2002 was £446 million, £31 million more than in 2000–2001.

2 the elimination of litigation expenses (specifically, lawyers' professional fees) as an element in the cost of compensating victims, thus increasing the funds available for actual compensation and for health care in general.

These are the arguments most strongly and persistently put forward by parties such as the British Medical Association.[15] They are also the arguments behind the government's current thinking. For example, the announcement of the Donaldson consultation was accompanied by the statement:

> 'Reform is not about reducing compensation for patients. It is about ending the blame culture and, where possible, removing the burden of legal costs from the taxpayer.'[16]

The terms in which the debate on error prevention have been couched have been concerned with the elimination of the 'blame culture'. For example, the Department of Health paper *An Organisation with a Memory*[17] stated 'blame cultures … can encourage people to cover up errors for fear of retribution'. This perception appears frequently in the pages of the medical press[18–20]; and it is not held only in the UK. Phelan,[12] in discussing the opportunities for improvement in the quality of health care in Australia, writes:

> 'Identifying, investigating and responding to adverse events in a way that will limit their chance of recurrence is probably the single greatest opportunity for quality improvement. However, this requires a shift from a culture of blame to one that recognises such events as almost always a system failure.'

In February 2003, Professor Donaldson used a keynote address to a conference on patient safety to state that: 'serious medical errors are rarely solely the fault of individual healthcare workers but are the fault of the entire system'.[21]

It is the weight of these two arguments, therefore, which must be closely evaluated before fault is reformed or jettisoned as the criterion for compensation.

THE PRICE OF REFORM

Like most benefits, these two, if attainable, are likely to come with a price. There might be a variety of prices: financial, political, personal or ethical. Before we move, in the interests of a blame-free culture, to compensation by reference to criteria other than fault, we should consider the price for so doing and whether we are willing to pay it. A dispassionate examination of the issue forces us to the conclusion that the ethical price of radically reforming the present fault-based system of compensating those injured in the course of medical treatment will be substantial; further, it may not be worth paying, because the main benefits sought from such reform will probably not follow.

What we mean when we speak of an ethical price is, for example, the consideration that some errors may be so blameworthy that they ought not to escape notice and even punishment. It has been commented, even in the context of a pragmatic study of incident reporting for error avoidance, that '… we have to do something when we know there is a problem. Failure to do that could *and should* result in blame'[22] (emphasis added). There are other acts and omissions, too, which ought to result in blame. If blame is not attributed in these cases, we have lost something of value.

Ethical prices may be worth paying if the undoubtedly worthwhile benefits mentioned above can definitely be secured and if the loss can be limited. In this case, however, further consideration of the evidence compels us to doubt the certainty of the benefits and gives us grounds to fear the size of the potential loss.

DOUBTS ABOUT THE BENEFITS

Error reporting

The key service improvement mechanism arising from a blame-free culture must be an increase in the quantity and quality of error reporting; if we do not blame the person who commits the error, there is a greater chance of openness. The Donaldson consultation paper bluntly asserted: 'a no-fault system would also mean NHS staff would not have to be "blamed" for problems, encouraging a more open system'.[5]

But it does not take long to realise that for any clinical professional there are adverse consequences of a finding of fault, quite apart from possible legal liability, which are in themselves enough to prevent frank voluntary disclosure. Some of these adverse consequences are external and cultural; others are internal and psychological.

The external consequences do include blame, punishment and liability, but also loss of peer esteem, reduced career opportunities and the facing of difficult personal confrontations with colleagues and patients. The internal consequences include shame and guilt and these can be at least as powerful. Billings,[23] for example, found in a 1998 study that clinicians' reasons for non-reporting of error were: fear of embarrassment, punishment (of self or others) and litigation; and lack of belief in the likelihood of improvement.

Shame and guilt are both what psychologists call 'moral emotions'.[24,25] That is, they are capable of motivating consciously moral behaviour. There is, however, a psychological distinction between them.

Guilt is based on the actor's own values and is a motivator towards such behaviours as confession, apology and restitution; Eisenberg[25] typifies it as follows:

'The guilty actor accepts responsibility for a behaviour that violates internal standards and causes another's distress and desires to make amends.'

Shame, by contrast, is based on what others think of the actor and consequently is a powerful motivator of silence and concealment. To quote Eisenberg again[25]:

'The ashamed person ... feels self-conscious about the visibility of one's actions, fears scorn and avoids or hides from others ...'

In the context of clinical error, this tendency is probably exacerbated by the selection and conditioning of health professionals, particularly doctors, for perfectionism. Leape[26] says:

'the worst punishments are often self-inflicted: shame and guilt. The expectation of perfect performance is deeply ingrained in doctors and nurses, beginning in school and then with continual reinforcement in everyday practice. Shame results when we fail, which we inevitably do. Not surprisingly, physicians and nurses often will not admit errors – to themselves or others. They don't report errors they can hide.'

Benbasset et al's[9] study of medical attitudes to error also found a consistent theme of fear of personal inadequacy and failure among medical students and qualified physicians.

Negligence litigation carries the fear of exposure and shame. Even prior to litigation, the issue of error reporting is distorted by such fears. A recent editorial on error reporting in two leading journals[24,27] asks:

'who can doubt that the real agenda in the controversy currently raging over mandatory reporting of medical errors is the fear of being shamed?'

and concludes that

'shame is a powerful force in slowing or preventing improvement'.

The psychological literature identifies a range of possible reactions to critical incidents by those responsible. This range is described by Benbasset et al,[9] in a study of attitudes towards uncertainty and medical error, as:

1 personal acceptance of responsibility and seeking constructive change
2 denial – the repression of mistakes by forgetting or 'blanking out'
3 discounting – the blaming of others (the system, colleagues or the patient)
4 distancing – impersonal acceptance ('it was unavoidable').

A further factor noted in this and other studies is a positive correlation between fear of litigation, on the one hand and, on the other, strong support for self-regulation and resistance to involvement of others in the system of accountability.

It is, therefore, striking but not surprising to note Lawton and Parker's finding in a study carried out in 1998,[28] that doctors in particular (far more than nurses or midwives) are reluctant to report adverse incidents, even those which not only involve a breach of protocol but also result in harm to a patient. This, they suggest, goes some way to explain the widely documented[29] under-reporting of error.

Within the NHS, these reactions are so common and so tacitly understood that a group of forty senior clinicians, asked in 2000 to list the 'unwritten rules' by which the system actually runs, included in a long list:

'Anonymity confers mutual protection.
Only someone of my profession understands my problem.
Don't admit to mistakes.

It is wrong to be wrong …
… and it is wrong to admit to being wrong'.[30]

Cost reduction

There is also evidence that the second proposed benefit of replacing fault, the reduction of cost, may be as hard to deliver. That this evidence is overwhelming is convincingly shown in the analysis of the options in *Making Amends*.

The best recent summaries of reliable facts about the financial costs of clinical negligence litigation are probably the reports of the NAO. The following points can be drawn from their April 2001 report *Handling Clinical Negligence Claims in England*.[8]

The annual cost to the NHS of provision for claims rose from 1995/6 to 2000/1 by a factor of seven.[ii] This was so in spite of the fact that many people with grounds to claim compensation for fault do not do so, either because they do not know they can (the Department of Health does not currently believe the NHS has a public duty to tell patients when there may be evidence of negligence in their treatment – a position which *Making Amends* proposed should be replaced by an explicit duty of candour) or because they can not afford to.

Of these two natural brakes on the growth of litigation, affordability is likely to become an increasingly significant bar to claims, because the government intends to withdraw public funding for clinical negligence cases[31] and has for some time been raising the means threshold for eligibility and limiting the number of law firms who may handle cases. The number of legally aided cases alleging clinical negligence peaked in 1995/6 at 13 366. By 2000/1 this had fallen to 6197, less than half that for the previous year. The overall success rate in clinical negligence claims was found to be 24%.[32]

The government's policy is to reduce the legal aid budget by encouraging claimants to use 'no win, no fee' arrangements. In these, the solicitors finance the claim in the hope of receiving an enhanced success fee; this has the obvious result of further inflating the cost of successful claims by the success fee. The legal aid budget is thus relieved, but at the expense of the NHS compensation budget – a singular absence of joined-up thinking.

Clinical negligence cases are, of course, characterised by the inherent uncertainty of issues of diagnosis, prognosis and causation; their outcome is, consequently, hard to predict. In the absence of a National Justice Service, modelled on the National Health Service, offering legal representation by salaried public employees free at the point of delivery, potential claimants must seek representation from private practitioners. These have to price their services, like pre-NHS doctors, at a level to afford themselves a living. It is difficult to argue that solicitors in private practice are under a duty to fund all

---

[ii]Of course, as has already been noted, there has been a considerable rise in provision since this report, largely because of changed actuarial projections.

uncertain claims from their own pockets on principle *pro bono publico* (unless, like some, one believes that all solicitors are automatically wealthy 'fat cats').[iii] Hence, the NAO concluded in 2001[8] that patients do not currently have access to mechanisms that will deliver appropriate resolutions to their problems in a timely and efficient way. This conclusion was far less widely reported than the same report's findings as to the global costs of negligence litigation to the NHS.

We should also note that a very high proportion, by value, of claims (either 80%, according to the NAO[8] or 60% according to *Making Amends*)[33] are accounted for by a relatively small number of cases of catastrophic damage to infants. These claims are the hardest to shrug off as frivolous or lacking in merit. It is perhaps for this reason that *Making Amends* proposed an entirely separate compensation system for birth-related neurological damage.

Of course, clear and careful comparisons of any suggested new model with existing fault-based and no-fault compensation systems are needed and this requires empirical research, which is not the object of this chapter. Fortunately, however, the longstanding interest in no-fault compensation has led to a number of studies based on empirical data and the existence of at least four countries, Sweden, Norway, Finland and New Zealand which have adopted such systems has made meaningful comparison possible. *Making Amends* discussed these systems and others at some length.

There is a distinct and natural tendency for those who carry out such comparisons to find what they want to find (whether for or against reform) and their conclusions need to be considered with care. However, one indication from the data they offer is that where cost savings have actually been achieved, it has been done by two strategies: restricting the range of events giving eligibility for compensation; and limiting levels of compensation to those injured.[34]

One particularly interesting study is that of Studdert and Brennan[35]: this is unapologetically in favour of the introduction of no-fault compensation on the Swedish model to replace the malpractice litigation system in the USA. The authors reach this conclusion largely by arguing that there is an inherent and unavoidable conflict between error prevention and the tort system. They address the issue of comparative financial cost head on, by calculating compensation on three bases: (i) compensation of all adverse events; (ii) compensation of events compensable under the Swedish system (broadly defined as 'avoidable'); and (iii) compensation of fault-based events.

Their immediate finding is that the introduction of the Swedish system in the USA would increase global compensation costs by an average of 50%. This

---

[iii] In 2001, the Law Society quoted the average (mean) gross fees (i.e. before expenses) per solicitor in private practice as ranging from £68 000 for sole practitioners to £159 000 for firms with 26 or more partners (Key facts 2001: the Solicitors' Profession. London: The Law Society; 2001). In October 2002 Sheffield Careers Guidance Service was advising those who consulted its website that average gross earnings for a solicitor were around £39 000 p.a. (Online. Available: http://www.scgs.org.uk/careerslegal.htm 31 Oct 2002.)

is a striking conclusion from enthusiasts for no-fault, in the country where malpractice litigation is most widely represented as running out of control and which should therefore presumably present most opportunity to save money by eliminating litigation costs.

In the light of this finding, the authors' judgement, realistically enough, is that:

'States cannot reasonably be expected to pilot no-fault schemes, much less adopt them, if their costs will significantly exceed those of the current malpractice system.'[35]

Their proposed solution, therefore, is what they call '*practical* versions of a Swedish style scheme' (emphasis added). In this context, 'practical' means, inevitably, a reduced class eligible for compensation and/or reduced payment tariffs. This is further developed in a subsequent paper by Studdert and Brennan,[36] which discusses in detail where to set the threshold for eligibility and how to fix the compensation package.

Making Amends was compelled to conclude that a full-blooded no-fault system offered the prospect of more claims and increased expense.

One point which stands out in studies of this sort is that the link between penalisation of fault and behavioural change is represented as a simple pragmatic/financial one: the clinician is assumed to think, clearly and simply, 'I have made an error; if I report it, I may be sued; I had better keep quiet'; or else 'if I report it, I will not be blamed/sued and we may learn how to avoid future errors; I will report it'. This picture is grossly simplistic; it fails, it is submitted, to describe accurately the real and complex moral and psychological interaction involved in error reporting.

Ethical costs of reform

In the end, we might decide that the financial cost of a no-fault system must be borne, for the operational benefits it may bring. However, the cost of replacing fault is ethical as well as financial.

In spite of Studdert and Brennan's enthusiasm for no-fault systems, they recognise one serious ethical objection to cost saving by systems designed to encourage 'under-claiming', namely that it raises serious questions of fairness. This has deeper implications, including political ones.

The New Labour government's argument in its 2002 Budget for general taxation as the way to pay for quality health care contained a significant ethical component. We should pay through general taxation, it was argued, because this is the *fairest* way.[37] If another system (e.g. insurance based) were less expensive but less fair, that would be a reason to reject it. In other words, some systems have an ethical deficit, in terms of justice, which should make us hesitate before adopting them.

This position is a powerful one, both philosophically and politically. It may be unjust (unfair, if you prefer that term) to cease to require those in breach of duty directly to compensate those injured in consequence. This ethical cost has a number of components, of which three will be dealt with here, namely:

1 a loss of *accountability*, by the severance of the link between substandard performance and a formal, public, finding of fault (which may be of great significance for those harmed by poor performance);
2 a loss of *equality* of treatment, by an increased discrepancy in the answerability of different professional groups for their standards of performance; and
3 most seriously, an explicit acceptance that unethical behaviour by medical professionals – that is, the *concealment* of error, in order to avoid adverse personal consequences – is inevitable unless amnesty is offered.

Accountability

Accountability has become a popular word in public discourse, largely because it is a concept by which central government may justify increased inspection of, and explicit prescription of standards for, all parts of the public and quasi-public sector. Those in receipt of public funds in particular – in education, health, law enforcement and so on – are expected to account for their stewardship and to be answerable for substandard service provision. Paul Boateng, the then Health Minister, acknowledged this in Parliament in 1998 when, rejecting no-fault compensation, he said: 'There is a risk that a no-fault culture could, over time, diminish clinical accountability'.[38] The concept has given birth, in the health sector alone, to a number of bodies, of which CHI and NPSA are two.

Mr Boateng also argued that 'to pay compensation when no fault has been established would, to some extent, belittle the harm caused to others through a negligent act'.[39] The reaction of those who, or whose loved ones, have suffered harm, is instructive. Whether in Bristol, Alder Hey, North Staffordshire or elsewhere, there is a clear desire that those who have failed to meet professional standards should be in some way answerable, that is, experience some formal pronouncement of responsibility and not simply to walk away. The fact of *informal* adverse personal consequences (bad publicity, professional disadvantage) is not the point. A public ruling as to why, how, by whose fault, this has happened appears to be part of the process of coming to terms with the harm.

This is sometimes represented as a vindictive desire to see another suffer, too, and this may indeed be present in some cases. But the frequently remarked effectiveness of a prompt and unqualified apology is one indicator that to paint a picture of negligence claimants as simply vindictive gold-diggers is a drastic misrepresentation of a complex set of psychological responses.

Professional inequality

An immediate problem for any medical professional supporting the radical replacement of the clinical negligence system is that arguments on behalf of any group that they should be exempt from legal liability for their actions have a tendency to appear self-serving. A conflict of interest is unavoidable. This does not necessarily mean that the argument for reform is without merit, but it is surprising to note that some of the keenest proponents of abolition are prepared to argue that the fear of litigation may be salutary for others, such as trusts and managers, though not for their own professional group.

Any compensation system has, of course, to include some limiting factors to keep the 'floodgates of litigation' in check, but some of these can, in the long term, prove counter-productive. Limiting the recovery of compensation, on pragmatic grounds, against one group of professionals, while permitting it in analogous circumstances against others, sets up a conflict within the system and is ethically questionable in terms of justice – surely the primary principle expected to be exemplified by the legal system. This, too, was implicitly present in Mr Boateng's argument in 1998 when he said:

> 'When an adverse effect is the result of third party misconduct or negligence, it is right that the harmed person should be able to seek some recompense. The underlying principles … apply to personal injury cases in general, not just those arising from health care. *We are not persuaded that health care should be singled out for different treatment*' [emphasis added].[39]

An example of this in case law is the way in which the judges treat doctors differently from, say, surveyors, solicitors or auditors. The *Bolam* principle (*Bolam v. Friern Hospital Management Committee* [1957] 1 WLR 582) permits the opinion of a body of doctors to set the standard by which it will be determined whether one of their number is in breach of the duty of care. This standard is then accepted by the court as definitive, even if it is not accepted by a majority of doctors and even if experience since the date of the incident in question has shown it to be deficient. The only exception, rarely if ever applied in practice, is when the opinion is found logically indefensible (*Bolitho (deceased) v. City and Hackney Health Authority* [1998] AC 232).

In a contrasting example, the courts have ruled that it was negligent for a conveyancing solicitor to comply with the universally accepted practice of conveyancers in the market because, with hindsight, his client was harmed by it (*Edward Wong Finance Co Ltd. v. Johnson, Stokes and Master* [1984] AC 296). Judges are no more conveyancers than they are doctors, but they can, apparently, assess the standard of care for the conveyancer, while steadfastly refusing to second-guess the doctor.

The criticism of inequality can legitimately be levelled at the current clinical negligence system, which provides greater protection for doctors, through the *Bolam* rule and other mechanisms, than for any other professional group. This inequality would be enormously increased by the effective abolition of fault liability for health professionals and its retention for others.

Acceptance of concealment

The heaviest ethical price of abolishing fault, it was suggested above, is the pragmatic acceptance that doctors will cover up – even lie – rather than admit error and that no law, no professional code and no personal conscience can be expected to change this. To return to error reporting systems, should we simply accept that the concealment of fault is inevitable, or ought we to deem this ethically unacceptable behaviour in itself – to err being human, but to cover up being unforgivable? What, if any, actions intended to avoid responsibility for our faults are justifiable?

The ethical inadequacy of accepting self-protecting concealment behaviour as inevitable, on a sort of 'boys will be boys' argument, must be clear to any thoughtful observer. One has only to observe the criticism levelled at any person or body who is suspected of involvement in a cover-up to conclude that there is broad consensus on this in our society. To what extent, therefore, ought we to structure our compensation mechanisms, with a despairing shrug, on the basis that those who have failed to meet professional standards, or whose actions have contributed to harm to others, will allow this to become known only if they are offered personal amnesty?

Further, this argument is insulting to the many doctors who, when they make an error (as all may from time to time), frankly admit the fact, whatever the personal consequences, and do everything in their power to recompense anyone harmed by their conduct.

CONCLUSION

To summarise the argument so far, the objections to the 'no blame/no fault' proposal are that it will prove to be either expensive or unfair, that it is psychologically unrealistic and that in the final analysis it may be morally repugnant.

This is disappointing, to say the least of it. It should lead us, however, to some more fundamental questions, which may either lead us to design a system better than the one we have at present, or else to conclude that the current system, with less radical adjustments, is the best we can come up with to achieve the variety of ends which our society has in view for it.

We need a more radical analysis of compensation systems – what they seek to achieve, how they seek to achieve it and why that particular basis of compensation is chosen. The fundamental question to answer in any process of reform is: What is the necessary ethical, as distinct from causative, link between substandard health care and financial compensation?

Will the simple *need* of the patient suffice? Non-fault compensation systems clearly go beyond need. At the very least, they seek to compensate avoidable injury. Unavoidable or random injury goes uncompensated.

Why, in any case, do we talk in terms of 'compensation' for the victims of adverse outcomes? Why do we not just treat everyone according to need, regardless of the cause of need? After all, a patient such as a driver injured in a road traffic accident is treated alike, regardless of whether the injury has been caused by another's fault, the driver's own fault or sheer misadventure. This is especially true in the NHS, based on health care delivered free *at the point of need*. So why should we treat those whose loss is caused by a breach of a healthcare professional's duty differently from the victims of accident or disease?

We ought to consider why we give lump-sum financial payments to those injured by another's fault, but provide for the needs of those injured or sick without fault by means of income payments through the benefit system and health care through the NHS. The logic of no-fault compensation, if carried to its logical conclusion, is that no private individual should get compensation for any injury, medical or otherwise: rather, the state will provide for them through a needs-related (and hence, presumably, a means-tested) benefit system; and the state will, where deemed appropriate on policy grounds, recover the resulting cost from anyone at fault. The resources hitherto put into compensating those harmed through negligence would, instead, be diverted into the general health and social care systems, to enable them better to care for the victims of avoidable medical error along with all others in need.

To realise that this is more than a theoretical possibility, we need go no further than the consultations held by the Lord Chancellor's Department in March 2000 and March 2002[40,41] to consider alternatives to lump sum awards in personal injury actions. The suggestion that there should be 'structured settlements' for the catastrophically injured, involving periodical payments and non-financial provision, is in any case not new. The NAO, in its 2001 report,[8] commended the 'package' approach to compensation, which sees it as 'an extension of care rather than just as a legal process'. If compensation is part of care, why should it be offered in a form not offered to others whose needs are just as great?

The answer must be a *moral* link between fault and compensation.

These ethical and other costs need to be borne in mind when we balance the pros and cons of replacement of fault as the basis for compensation. The removal of the duty/breach element from the error compensation system presents us with a significant justice deficit. It is submitted that any no-fault scheme must overcome this deficit, if it is to be an improvement.

In summary, if the current system is defective and the proposed alternative ethically unacceptable in a society concerned to hold accountable those to whom it entrusts responsibility, what, so to speak, is Plan C? Until we can confidently answer this question, despite the enormous political and operational pressure to 'do something', the only safe conclusion is that we would be ill advised to remove fault as the essential link between error and compensation.

Afterword – *Making Amends*

Making Amends represents Professor Donaldson's Plan C. He has been one of the major individual enthusiasts for a no-blame culture and the NPSA has been perceived as his baby and the primary no-blame agency. His report, however, proposes what appear to be surprisingly modest amendments.

The main proposal is the establishment of an NHS Redress Scheme. This is intended to offer investigation, explanation, a 'package of care' and payments for certain harms (but not, apparently, loss of earnings) up to £30 000.

For claimants seeking more than this, their only option will remain the courts, but damages at law will not be based on the cost of private medical care; presumably the claimant will have to rely on the NHS for what it could provide. There will also be a 'presumption' that the claimant has first applied to the Scheme. Presumably this means that not doing so would count as a failure by the claimant to mitigate his/her loss, which would reduce damages and costs. Acceptance of a 'package' under the Scheme will involve waiver of the right to sue.

Neurologically impaired babies would be dealt with under a different scheme, but here too there would be a move away from one-off lump sum damages to care, monthly payments and capped capital payments.

The no-blame elements are to be a statutory exemption from disciplinary action for those who report errors and legal privilege for documents and information identifying adverse events. The *quid pro quo* would be a statutory duty of candour, to inform patients about actions which have caused harm (a real step forward for patients).

Questions of detail, of course, remain. For example, one criterion for payment under the Scheme is 'serious shortcomings in the standards of care'. It is left unclear how the appropriate standard is to be identified and how much lower a threshold this is than the legalistic *Bolam* test, which so favours clinical professionals and their employers.

The proposals have many positive aspects. In particular, they grasp for the first time the logic of a healthcare system which is meant to provide for our needs without payment and they recognise that, in practice, the response of clinicians to the risk of liability for error has been patterns of action which seek to avoid liability, rather than those which seek to eliminate error.

Looked at globally, the tone of *Making Amends* is sympathetic to clinical professionals and hostile to legal professionals (perhaps predictably, since the Chief Medical Officer is its author), most explicitly in the introduction to the all-important proposals for reform.[42] However, the most telling conclusion is that, even after recent reforms, the negligence system 'creates few incentives for providers of health care to reduce risk'.[43] It was surely this conclusion, above all, which convinced Professor Donaldson that negligence should be moved to 'the outer perimeter of the NHS'.[6]

What is less clear is that his modest proposals pass the test of ethics set out above, or that they justify any ethical price by being more effective than the blunt instrument of litigation in persuading clinicians to be open about error and so reach the Holy Grail of error prevention.

References

1 British Medical Association Parliamentary Unit. No fault compensation for medical injuries. London: BMA; 2001.
2 Hansard, 8 April 1998: cols 456–458.
3 Kennedy I. Learning from Bristol: The report of the public inquiry into children's heart surgery at the Bristol Royal Infirmary 1984–1995. London: The Stationery Office; 2001.

4 Department of Health. Clinical negligence: what are the issues and options for reform? London: The Stationery Office; 2001.

5 Donaldson L. Making amends. A consultation paper setting out proposals for reforming the approach to clinical negligence in the NHS. London: The Stationery Office; 2003.

6 Donaldson L. Making amends. A consultation paper setting out proposals for reforming the approach to clinical negligence in the NHS. London: The Stationery Office; 2003:119, para 10.

7 NHS (England) Summarised Accounts 2001–2002. London: National Audit Office; 2003.

8 National Audit Office. Handling clinical negligence claims in England. London: NAO; 2001.

9 Benbasset J, Pilpel D, Schor R. Physicians' attitudes towards litigation and defensive practice: development of a scale. Behavioural Medicine 2001; 27(2):52–61.

10 Passmore K, Leung W-C. Defensive practice among psychiatrists: a questionnaire survey. Postgraduate Medical Journal 2002; 78:671–673.

11 Donaldson L. In: Hargreaves S. 'Weak' safety culture behind errors, says chief medical officer. British Medical Journal 2003; 326(7384):300.

12 Phelan P. Improving the quality of health-care: personal reflections on some opportunities and impediments. Journal of Quality in Clinical Practice 2001; 21:34–36.

13 Donaldson L. Making amends. A consultation paper setting out proposals for reforming the approach to clinical negligence in the NHS. London: The Stationery Office; 2003:117, para 3.

14 Vincent C, Neale G, Woloshynowych M. Adverse incidents in British hospitals: preliminary retrospective record review. British Medical Journal 2001; 322:517–519.

15 British Medical Association Parliamentary Unit. No fault compensation for medical injuries. London: BMA; 2001.

16 Ananova, 7 July 2001.

17 Department of Health. An organisation with a memory. London: The Stationery Office; 2000.

18 Nottingham J. Perhaps blame-free culture is needed in NHS to reduce errors. British Medical Journal 2001; 322:1421.

19 Hall D. No blame should be apportioned in corporate failure. British Medical Journal 2001; 323:1130.

20 Wise J. UK government and doctors agree to end 'blame culture'. British Medical Journal 2001; 323:9.

21 Hargreaves S. 'Weak' safety culture behind errors, says chief medical officer. British Medical Journal 2003; 326(7384):300.

22 Wilson T, Haraden C. Words, words and more words. Clinical Governance Bulletin 2001; 2(5):13.

23 Billings C. Some hopes and concerns regarding medical event-reporting systems. Archives of Pathology and Laboratory Medicine 1998: 122:214–215, cited in: Leape L. Reporting of medical errors: time for a reality check. Western Journal of Medicine 2001; 174:159–161.

24 Davidoff F. Shame: the elephant in the room. Quality and Safety in Health Care 2002; 11:2–4.

25 Eisenberg N. Emotion, regulation and moral development. Annual Review of Psychology 2000; 51:665–697.

26 Leape L. Reporting of medical errors: time for a reality check. Western Journal of Medicine 2001; 174:159–161.

27   Davidoff F. Shame: the elephant in the room. British Medical Journal 2002; 324:623–624.

28   Lawton R, Parker D. Barriers to incident reporting in a healthcare system. Quality and Safety in Health Care 2002; 11:15–18.

29   Woods D. Estimate of 98 000 deaths from medical errors is too low, says specialist. British Medical Journal 2000; 320:1362.

30   Cullen R, Nicholls S, Halligan A. Reviewing a service – discovering the unwritten rules. British Journal of Clinical Governance 2000; 5(4):233–239.

31   Slapper G. Litigation, publically funded law, CPS Report, Justice for All. Student Law Review 2002; 37:27–31.

32   Dobson R. Legally aided medical negligence cases fall sharply. British Medical Journal 2001; 322:1018.

33   Donaldson L. Making amends. A consultation paper setting out proposals for reforming the approach to clinical negligence in the NHS. London: The Stationery Office; 2003:47.

34   Dewees D, Duff D, Trebilcock M. Exploring the domain of accident law: taking the facts seriously, 1996. In: Kennedy I, Grubb A, eds. Medical law: text with materials. London: Butterworths; 2000.

35   Studdert D, Brennan T. No-fault compensation for medical injuries: the prospect for error prevention. Journal of the American Medical Association 2001; 286(2):217.

36   Studdert D, Brennan T. Towards a workable model of 'no-fault' compensation for medical injury in the United States. American Journal of Law & Medicine 2000; 27:225–252.

37   Hansard, 17 April 2002: col. 591.

38   Hansard, 8 April 1998: col. 457.

39   Hansard, 8 April 1998: col. 456.

40   Lord Chancellor's Department. Damages: the discount rate and alternatives to lump sum payments. London: The Stationery Office; 2000.

41   Lord Chancellor's Department. Damages for future loss: giving the courts the power to order periodical payments for future loss and care costs in personal injury cases. London: The Stationery Office; 2002.

42   Donaldson L. Making amends. A consultation paper setting out proposals for reforming the approach to clinical negligence in the NHS. London: The Stationery Office; 2003:117–119.

43   Donaldson L. Making amends. A consultation paper setting out proposals for reforming the approach to clinical negligence in the NHS. London: The Stationery Office; 2003:118, para 9.

Chapter 5

Creating a level playing field? The influence of user and provider grievances in the shaping of healthcare policy

Susan Kerrison

TIPPING THE BALANCE TOWARDS USERS

The NHS plan attempts to give users greater influence over the way publicly funded services are provided by both public and private sectors.[1] The aim is to create a level playing field between service users and providers. But this chapter argues that the different arrangements for handling complaints and grievances from private providers and users, give the former privileged influence over policy. Formal legal rights of influence come about in three ways: through the ballot box, through representations to the courts and through 'quasi legal' procedures such as grievance procedures or complaints handling. Thus law determines who can speak and whether or not service providers are required to pay attention. English law treats both users of health care and private providers as private citizens but affords them different rights to be heard. Users have rights through the ballot box and the courts but only weak procedures for complaint.[2,3] In contrast, the appeals systems and grievance procedures available to private providers, designed to constrain the discretion of public officials, allow private providers greater influence in decision making.

In the UK healthcare system, public and private providers are now regulated. But the arrangements for handling complaints and grievances against regulators mean that there is a potential for private providers to have greater influence over the regulator's policies. With the emergence of a mixed economy of providers, there are now good reasons for rethinking the balance between the private citizen and the private provider. In other sectors, such as utilities, different arrangements for grievance handling have evolved, suggesting that legal devices which tip the balance towards the user can be designed. Moreover, these have proved an aid to the regulatory task.[4,5] As such a framework has not been employed in the healthcare sector, the influence of government and providers has been maintained at the expense of users – a situation which may make the task of healthcare regulators more difficult.

Recent UK healthcare policy is marked by a search for new institutional forms to replace the old idea of services delivered by the NHS under the control of the Department of Health. Private sector providers have been encouraged to the extent that in 1999, over 50% of all healthcare beds[i] in the UK were in the private sector. Plans for the introduction of semi-autonomous foundation hospital trusts have also been developed.[6] 'Arms length' intermediary bodies or regulatory agencies such as the new Commission for Healthcare Audit and Inspection (CHAI) have been charged with the task of ensuring the quality of care in this network of semi-autonomous public and private providers.[7] But influence over the decision-making processes is unequal because of differing access to power and resources between government, public and private providers and users.

With this type of networked structure, the governance of the UK healthcare sector now shares much in common with other regulated sectors of the economy such as utilities or financial services. But as with other sectors, the notional independence of the regulatory agency is often illusory.[4,5] On the one hand, the government tends to maintain significant powers over the agency or key functions within the sector. On the other hand, as regulation of private sector companies requires a legal framework, important areas of policy are opened up for determination by the legal system. For the first time, law becomes involved in a significant way in healthcare policy. In this system, policy making tends to become fragmented between government, regulators and the legal system while government intent is refracted through regulatory agencies, courts and appeal tribunals. Thus, the policy-making process is altogether less transparent and less amenable to parliamentary or democratic control.

---

[i]NHS beds available in England in 1999 – 179 000, data from 'Bed availability and occupancy in England', Department of Health, published annually. Beds in private or independent hospitals or nursing homes 202 000, data from 'Community care statistics' Department of Health, published annually.

Given this situation, there have been calls within public law for the development of an extended notion of accountability to cope better with this transformation in public services.[8] For example, Prosser[9] argues that regulation is in effect 'government in miniature' and therefore procedures such as grievance procedures should be developed which more fully incorporate consumer interests. Complaints systems and grievance handling have been bound up with the constitutional status of the institutions providing health care.[3] The nature of these institutions is now changing with concurrent changes in the characteristics of such grievance procedures.

THE COMPLAINTS SYSTEM 1996 TO 2003 – MAINTAINING THE SOVEREIGNTY OF PARLIAMENT AND THE AUTHORITY OF GOVERNMENT

The complaints system evolved in a ramshackle way to take account of the different constitutional status of the public and private sectors in English law. In an attempt to maintain the sovereignty of parliament, the system was essentially hidebound by this framework, granting users few legal rights of influence or challenge.[3] Between 1996 and 2003 there were essentially three different systems in operation: the NHS complaints system introduced in 1996, the Health Service Commissioner or Ombudsman and the regulators for private sector and healthcare professions. These three systems had differing jurisdictions and powers, labyrinthine in their complexity.[10] Like other systems in the UK public sector, it was difficult to view the procedures as having influence as they were all fettered in some way by outmoded legal frameworks.[10]

The NHS procedure, which dealt with complaints against the NHS providers and complaints against private providers funded by the NHS, was a two-stage process. The first stage consisted of an informal dispute resolution process. The second stage, a hearing before a panel whose independence was questionable could only be invoked if a 'convenor' agreed. As Mulcahy and Allsop commented,[11] complainants trying to raise issues of public concern were seen to be hindered at every threshold by discretionary powers granted to state agents to decide whether the issue ought to be pursued. The NHS procedure was so informal, so internal to the service and so lacking in procedural constraints that a national evaluation[12] found that the majority of complainants were dissatisfied and perceived the procedure as biased towards that service.

After the NHS procedure was exhausted, complainants had a right of appeal to the Health Ombudsman. The Ombudsman or Health Service Commissioner is an officer of parliament whose function is to provide in-depth investigations. Consequently, the Ombudsman only dealt with relatively few cases. In 2001–2002, the Health Service Ombudsman began investigations on 204 new cases[13] – a small figure for a health service for more than 59 million people. As there was only a small chance of any NHS written complaint being investigated (1 in 700 in 2000–2001),[14] the impact on the service was questionable. The Ombudsman could neither question nor criticise the merits of decisions taken without maladministration: instead the role was one of investigating and reporting to the Parliamentary Select Committee for Public Administration. The Ombudsman's powers were designed to maintain the sovereignty of Parliament and to protect the state from any challenge to its policies.[15,16] Yet, parliamentary sovereignty was becoming an increasing fiction, with the Select Committee also lacking any real control over the NHS. For example, in 1998 it commented:

> 'This Committee's predecessors have made recommendations relating to the management of the NHS almost every year since 1976. Nevertheless, year after year, the results of investigations by the Ombudsman reveal the same failings. Our predecessors wrote in 1996 that despite the circulation of the Ombudsman's report within the NHS, in certain areas such as complaints handling, records management and dealing with bereavement there is as yet no obvious improvement. What we say in this report shows that this is still true.'[17]

While the regulatory agencies governing the private sector and the professions had an important role in handling complaints, they nevertheless lacked a legal mandate for general dispute resolution.[10] Without such a mandate they tended only to be interested in a complaint if it indicated a breach in regulatory rules. Complainants were thus cast into the role of public spirited individuals reporting a problem rather than citizens with a grievance attempting to hold a provider to account. For some agencies, complaints had a low priority. For example, the Human Fertilisation and Embryology Authority did not set up a complaints procedure until 2002, over 10 years after its foundation. In the case of private care homes, the Office of Fair Trading[18] found that complainants were very dissatisfied with the way that the regulated agencies, health authorities and local authorities handled complaints about homes. Some investigations were conducted without reference to the complainant and in others the findings were notified to the person or body against whom the complaint was made ahead of the complainant. Regulatory agencies were thus open to criticisms that they were not responsive to users and that it was difficult to see the complaints process as a vehicle for raising issues of wider public concern.

Yet, in terms of influencing policy, there were even more fundamental problems with these arrangements. There was no link between those bodies that had authority over the NHS – the Commission for Health Improvement, the Audit Commission, the NHS Executive or the Department of Health – and the complaints procedures. With no right of appeal to or involvement in such governing agencies, the findings of complaints enquiries were unlikely to have any effect on those charged with policy development or its enforcement.

A NEW STRUCTURE FOR UK HEALTH CARE TAKES SHAPE

While the old complaints system was a creature of the old model of health care, by 2002 a new shape for the sector was solidifying. A new legal framework for the regulation of the private healthcare sector, the Care Standards Act 2000, had been introduced. This Act also established a new commission – the National Care Standards Commission – to take over responsibilities for regulating private health care and the care sector in general from health authorities and local authorities. Reforms were also announced in the NHS complaints system, the public sector Ombudsman[19] and for management of the public sector. *Delivering the NHS Plans: The Next Steps*[20] indicated that the Commission for Health Improvement would be renamed the Commission for Healthcare Audit and Inspection (CHAI) and given new responsibilities. Equipped with new powers, the new Commission would take on a broader role, regulating quality standards in both the public and private sectors and would provide an independent review of complaints.[21] CHAI would also take over responsibility from the short-lived National Care Standards Commission for enforcing the provisions of the Care Standards Act in relation to private health care. CHAI would therefore have responsibilities across the whole healthcare sector, public and private, for ensuring that providers operated according to legal rules and government policies in the areas of quality of care, environment and value for money.[7]

The NHS Reform and Healthcare Professions Act 2002 further spelt out CHAI public sector functions. The Commission would be responsible for (1) setting standards in partnership with the Department of Health, (2) audit and inspection of performance, clinical governance and finance, (3) encouraging improvements in service delivery and (4) working with strategic health authorities to enforce standards. To ensure compliance and to encourage improvement, the new Commission has been given powers to recommend franchised management, suspension, or closure of any public provider found wanting. For the private sector, the provisions of the Care Standards Act 2000 require CHAI to register and set conditions for registration and inspections of all private providers, ensuring that they operate according to regulatory rules. The sanctions for non-compliance for private sector providers are withdrawal of their licence to operate and prosecution, which may result in a fine.

The NHS Reform Act also contained a major programme for strengthening public involvement in public health care including the provision for a Commission for Patient and Public Involvement (CPPI). The task of CPPI will be to promote user involvement and to oversee the new patient forums and the new Independent Complaints Advocacy Service (ICAS). The latter will be responsible for supporting all publicly funded complainants. The Commission for Patient and Public Involvement has a duty to advise the Secretary of State for Health on the arrangements for public involvement, and also report to CHAI issues of concern. However, the Act did not place any legal duty on CHAI to provide an independent review of user complaints.

This new structure for health care, of a regulator linked to an agency whose central concern is representing users or consumers, is similar to the approach adopted for the utilities sector.[4,5] The Utilities Act 2000 required the establishment of a consumer agency 'Energywatch'. The remit of 'Energywatch' is to 'have regard' to the interests of vulnerable consumers, to investigate any matter relating to the interests of consumers, to publish information on complaints and other matters in the consumer interest and to give advice to ministers. 'Energywatch' also has a duty to investigate and seek to resolve complaints from consumers in both the gas and electricity industries.

As no legal duty has currently been placed on CHAI to provide an independent review of complaints, the way is open for either CHAI or, adopting the utilities model, CPPI, to assume responsibility for independent review. However, the use of a consumer organisation to handle complaints in utilities is new and experience is limited.[4,5] The initial concern has been that the volume of complaints could overwhelm the consumer organisation, making it difficult for the organisation to carry out its other functions of representing consumers. There is, however, considerable experience of regulatory agencies dealing with complaints. Given that the intent was for CHAI to provide an independent complaints review, the dynamics and legal constraints on grievance handling by CHAI are analysed in the next section.

INFLUENCES AND LEGAL CONSTRAINTS ON THE INTERPRETATION OF REGULATORY RULES

Oversight of the complaints process by CHAI would be a major step forward. The first stage, informal resolution at the level of providers, would remain. But for the first time for public providers, there would be a second stage, which would provide an independent review of user complaints from an organisation with oversight of providers.

Regulators operate by ensuring that the providers comply with rules, which in the case of CHAI will be made by the Department of Health. Oversight of the complaints process can provide a means of monitoring compliance. Complaints can also be used to identify areas of potential concern and to provide evidence about the underlying cause of non-compliance. But all rules are inherently indeterminate.[22] Even the tightest of numerical standards needs interpretation and that interpretation can generally be disputed. Other rules may be deliberately framed vaguely, so that contentious areas are left open for negotiation.[23] For example, despite evidence[24] to suggest that staffing levels are directly linked to the quality of care, no minimum standards have been set for staffing levels in private hospitals or nursing homes.[23] Thus,

> 'The registered person shall, having regard to the nature of the establishment of agency and the number and needs of patients, ensure that there is at all times an appropriate number of suitably qualified, skilled and experienced persons employed in or for the purposes of the establishment ... '
>
> (Reg 18 (1) Statutory Instruments 2001 no 3968. Public Health England. The Private and Voluntary Health Care (England) Regulations 2001)

The meaning of 'appropriate' will have to be negotiated with each healthcare provider and will be subject to changes in patients' needs. So although the Commission is not required to frame regulatory rules, rules must nevertheless be interpreted in their application. In a sense, regulatory rules are made jointly, not only by legislatures but also by the recurrent actions of regulatory agencies, enforcement officials and all others who have a major influence on the behaviour of the agency and its officials.[25,26]

Regulation is acknowledged as inherently a matter of balancing the competing interests of, on the one hand, providers and, on the other hand, users, together with public interest. Public lawyers advocate procedures that would lead to greater explicitness and transparency in the way these interests are balanced,[4,5,8] for example, by placing a requirement on regulators to give evidence-based reasons for decisions. However, currently many influences on CHAI's interpretation of rules are opaque, particularly in relation to the public sector. It is hard to get an explicit picture of how and through what mechanism public sector providers will be controlled or, conversely, how they will influence policy and the interpretation of regulators' rules. Other influences are transparent because they are structured into the legal provisions. Thus the presence of legal constraints or the absence of duties on the agency, together with users' rights, make the intended balance between stakeholders clearer. This is explored in the next section.

Working under government instruction

The independence of regulatory agencies from government is one of the central issues which determines whether a regulator can decide its own policies and consequently, be responsive to the voices of users. The government has many ways of influencing the behaviour of agencies. For the public sector CHAI will remain a creature of the Department of Health. For the private sector, the Care Standards Act provides for direct intervention from the Department of Health. Section 6(2) enables the Secretary of State to instruct the Commission to act 'In accordance with any direction in writing given to it by the Secretary of State'. By contrast, the government may only directly interfere with utility regulators in very specific circumstances, for example, to maintain supply in extreme public emergencies such as war or natural disaster.[4,5] The Secretary of State for Health has already used the powers of intervention under the Care Standards Act to instruct the National Care Standards Commission, who currently regulate the private healthcare sector, to disapply the new space standards for rooms in nursing homes until 2007.[27] This suggests that no matter how open CHAI is, or no matter how fair its complaints procedures, its ability to respond to private sector users may be curtailed by government action. Users may be appealing to CHAI when it may be better for them to voice their concerns directly to government. Users who are unlikely to spend time reading statutes are presented with a confusing picture about where the power really lies.

The rights of providers – how large providers influence policy

Provisions may also be made for regulated providers to appeal against particular decisions of the regulator to an independent legal tribunal other than the courts.[28] Experience with other regulated industries and with old arrangements for nursing home regulation suggests that complaints to regulators from large corporate providers in particular, not only curb the regulators' freedom but also have an important effect in shaping regulatory policy.[29-31] Such providers are better organised and have more political, cultural, legal and economic resources to pursue their interest at appeal.

The provisions of the Care Standards Act empower CHAI to take administrative decisions, which can have a major effect on a private provider's business. CHAI can set conditions for registration affecting profitability or withdraw registration, so closing the provider's business. To guard against such draconian decisions being taken in an arbitrary manner, private providers have been given a right of appeal against these decisions. The traditional view is that this appeal system should be kept organisationally separate or independent from enforcement or rule making.[32] There are two reasons for this. First, it is suggested that where regulators act both as rule interpreter and adjudicator there is a risk of an institutional bias leading to a loss of the independence of mind required for adjudications. Second, fair adjudication is thought to be the application of existing standards. If regulatory agencies operate appeal systems, they may be inclined to allow other considerations or parties to be brought into play to produce a new interpretation. To guard against these problems, the Council on Tribunals has argued that appeal systems should have formal procedures and come under its supervision.[32] However, this tends to belie the fact that in practice it is difficult for tribunals to avoid making new interpretations of rules or even new rules. For example, the Registered Homes Tribunal resisted making rules on staffing levels in nursing homes for many years, but the agreements made by health authorities and providers as a result of a Tribunal decision nevertheless became the staffing standards for nursing homes.[33]

The Care Standards Act provides for an independent tribunal for appeals from the private providers, the Care Standards Tribunal (CST). Chaired by a lawyer and supervised by the Council on Tribunals, the CST hears appeals from registered persons on the conditions imposed on registration and on decisions by the regulator to withdraw registration. The CST has the power to take de novo decisions – that is to say it can substitute its decision for that of CHAI. Such arrangements have major disadvantages for regulatory agencies.[34] First, they tend to turn the Tribunal into the regulator and the regulator into the prosecutor. The problem is that interpretation of rules by bodies other than the regulator leads to inconsistencies. Baldwin and Cave,[35] drawing upon the empirical literature, suggest that the appeals procedure may increase delays and costs, destroy any policy cohesion in the regulatory agency and, if legalistic, may produce decisions which are less timely and less expert.

The second issue is that disputes around particular interpretation of rules can give rise to general issues of importance affecting the whole industry. But under the tribunal system such appeals are treated as though they only concerned the two parties, with intervention from expert witnesses only allowed. There are no procedural rights for users to be represented or their voices heard. Decisions are taken which affect the quality of the service provided to many users without any input from them or their representatives. Such disputes can also give rise to particular abuses of power, with large corporate providers bringing sufficient resources to bear in such disputes to tip the scales in their favour, skewing the rules for the whole industry. For example, under the Care Standards Tribunal predecessor, the Registered Homes Tribunal, an appeal by a major provider to this Tribunal was successful in setting the staffing pattern for large providers throughout the nursing home industry – despite its potential impact on residents.[33] While CHAI may hope to use complaints constructively to develop policy, its decisions may be overturned by CST. Policies re-enforced by the authority of a legal tribunal will not be so malleable to change as a result of appeals by users.

In contrast to the healthcare sector, utilities regulators have successfully resisted the argument from the Council on Tribunals for a separate process under the Council's supervision.[4,5,32] As there is no equivalent of the Care Standards Tribunal in the utilities sector, utilities regulators have significantly more control than CHAI over how the rules they enforce are interpreted. Under the Utilities Act 2000, utilities regulators only become involved in a small number of disputes which prove intractable or raise issues of general concern.[4,5] There is considerable evidence that utilities regulators will attempt to deal with issues of general concern by allowing parties other than those involved in a particular dispute to comment – either at a hearing or by calling for comments on a published draft decision.[4,5,32] In other words, unlike the closed nature of the tribunal process, the utility regulators have had the freedom to use the dispute resolution process openly, as a means of overt policy development.

In the case of the healthcare industry, complaints have been legally framed rather than dealt with as a process with a significant impact on policy. The Care Standards Tribunal was ostensibly set up to fulfil the traditional common law purpose described by Ogus as protecting 'individual rights against illegitimate government interference' where individuals are read as private providers.[36] A contemporary interpretation of the requirement to meet this purpose, based on human rights principles, would mean that interventions would be allowed from all parties who had an interest.[37,38] However, the arrangements for the Care Standards Tribunal takes no note of these changes. Neither do the arrangements take into account changes in the delivery of public services, which means that regulation is in effect 'government in miniature' and therefore requires procedures to incorporate users' interests more fully,[9] for example by allowing user groups the same standing as the regulatee to appeal the regulators' decision.[39] Where this does not occur, such tribunals are always at risk of capture by the industry.[39] CHAI's independence will be constrained by the Department of Health on the one hand, and by the decision of the Care Standards Tribunal on the other. The freedom of CHAI to act on the basis of user complaints, and hence the ability of the complaints to influence providers, will also be constrained by similar forces.

In the public sector CHAI will not be constrained by the decision of an appeals tribunal. It may have more freedom to determine its own interpretation of rules and the process of policy formation. However, as large foundation trusts with significant economic and legal resources begin to make use of their autonomy, there is a risk they will begin to exert pressure and challenge the regulator in an attempt to influence policy. The lack of procedural rules around grievance handling and policy formation will mean that the outcome of such interaction will be far from transparent. It would be valuable if in the public sector CHAI took a similar view to utilities regulators. Regulators in this sector have broadened out important disputes to examine the impact on, and allowed for comment from, all interested parties. Giving reasons for decisions based on evidence would also add to transparency.

The rights and influence of users

In practice, the legal framework currently constructed for CHAI does little to tip the balance towards users. Users have no rights of appeal to tribunals capable of overturning or examining the merits of CHAI decisions, other than the courts. Dissatisfied users may complain to the Parliamentary Commissioner for Administration (PCA). The PCA deals with complaints about all regulators, but these must be referred through an MP, and like other Ombudsmen, the PCA cannot examine the merits of a decision taken without maladministration. Currently this avenue is seldom used: a handful of complaints about all regulatory agencies have been received.[4,5] At the time of writing, the future role of the Health Ombudsman is unclear as it is under review.[19]

The consequence of the additional independent appeal procedures available to providers is to make the regulator unresponsive to users' complaints, particularly where the complaint would bring the regulator into conflict with large providers. It is not in the regulator's interest to be challenged by providers with large resources whose influence is attenuated by the procedural rights of appeal. A successful challenge would undermine the regulator's authority. Complainants are not homogeneous, and different procedures are available to different types of complainants – public or private providers or users. Users are not afforded the same procedural rights to intervene formally and challenge regulators' interpretation of rules as private providers. The presumption is that regulators operate in the public interest. While the intent may be to provide the same complaints review service irrespective of whether the user receives a service from a public or private provider, the fact that the policy drivers and legal and other constraints will be different for public and private sectors means that the dynamics of user influence is far from straightforward.

One further way of tipping the balance towards users is to ensure easy access to procedures for financial compensation or redress. The Ombudsman[13] has repeatedly argued for powers to insist that public providers financially compensate complainants, but these have not been forthcoming. In the case of publicly funded care, there are clearly arguments against this but where users pay for their own care then the objection is not clear cut. Utility regulators are empowered[4,5] to make determinations which have the force of county court judgments about terms and conditions of supply, compliance with terms and guaranteed standards, deposits and meter accuracy and billing disputes. But unlike utility regulators, CHAI has no powers to fine any providers for breaches in service provision or to insist on compensation or recompense. The lack of redress means that there is significant financial risk for people who fund their own care. For example, about a third of all nursing home residents, some 65 000 people, and the majority of those using fertility clinics receive no public funding. There is no provision to force private providers to provide recompense when there has been a clear breach of contract. For example, the fees for a private nursing home place may be in excess of £36 000 per year, yet if a private nursing home breaches its contract and does not provide adequate care, the residents or their relatives must sue the home for recompense rather than complain to the regulator with the expectation of financial redress. Not only would such a mechanism provide consumers who complain with a cheap alternative to the courts but it would also provide the regulator with a powerful additional sanction.

CONCLUSION

In practice, the potential of user complaints to influence CHAI's policy will depend on the freedom of the Commission to determine its own policies in the face of influence from both the government and providers. Few procedural rights have been granted to users which could balance the influence of these stakeholders. In the UK, provision of such rights tends to be unfavourably compared with the US system of rule and comment,[32] which is seen as procedural and legalistic. But a comparison with other UK sectors suggests it is possible to tip the balance more in favour of users without jeopardising the regulatory enterprise by collapsing into legalism. Indeed user rights can provide certain advantages to regulatory agencies.

However, this raises many difficult questions about the division of responsibility between central government and regulators. How is health policy to be determined? What is the balance between policies set by the regulators after a structured process involving many stakeholders, and those agreed by central government? As the Department of Health is a major purchaser of health care, such decisions could have a significant impact on public expenditure. This highlights a fundamental tension between, on the one hand, the independence of the regulator allowing responsiveness to users and reducing the risk of capture and, on the other hand, accountability to Parliament and the requirement to deliver a planned health service.

References

1 Department of Health. Involving patients and the public in health care: a discussion document. London: Department of Health; 2001.
2 Boyle AE. Sovereignty, accountability and the reform of administrative law. In: Richardson G, Genn H, eds. Administrative law and government action. Oxford: Clarendon Press; 1994.

3 Lewis N, Birkinshaw P. When citizens complain: reforming justice and administration. Buckingham: Open University Press; 1993.

4 Graham C. Regulating public utilities: a constitutional approach. Oxford: Hart; 2000.

5 Graham C. Is there a crisis in regulatory accountability? In: Baldwin R, Scott C, Hood C, eds. A reader on regulation. Oxford: Oxford University Press; 1998.

6 Department of Health. A guide to NHS foundation trusts. London: Department of Health; 2002.

7 Dewar S, Finlayson B. The I in the new CHAI. British Medical Journal 2002; 325: 848–850.

8 Scott C. Accountability in the regulatory state. Journal of Law and Society 2000; 27(1):38–60.

9 Prosser T. Law and the regulators. Oxford: Clarendon Press; 1997:305.

10 Kerrison SH, Pollock AM. Complaints as accountability: the case of health care in the UK. Public Law 2001; Spring:115–133.

11 Mulcahy L, Allsop J. A Woolf in sheep's clothing? Shifts towards informal resolution of complaints in the health service. In: Leyland P, Woods T, eds. Administrative law facing the future. Old constraints and new horizons. London: Blackstone; 1997:107–135.

12 Department of Health. NHS complaints procedure national evaluation. London: Department of Health; 2001.

13 The Health Service Ombudsman for England Annual Report 2001–2, HC 227. London: The Stationery Office; 2002.

14 Statistics from Department of Health. Handling complaints: monitoring the NHS complaints procedures England, financial year 2001–2. London: Department of Health; 2002.

15 Boyle AE. Sovereignty, accountability and the reform of administrative law. In: Richardson G, Genn H, eds. Administrative law and government action. Oxford: Clarendon Press; 1994:81–104.

16 Harlow C, Rawlings R. Law and administration. Oxford: Clarendon Press; 1997.

17 Select Committee on Public Administration Second Report 1997–8 HC 352 para 105. London: House of Commons; 1998.

18 Office of Fair Trading. Old people as consumers in care homes. London: OFT; 1998:242.

19 Collcutt P, Hourihan M. Review of the public sector Ombudsman in England. A report by the Cabinet Office; 2000.

20 Department of Health. Delivering the NHS plan: the next steps. London: Department of Health; 2002.

21 Department of Health. NHS complaints reform: making things right. London: Department of Health; 2003.

22 Black J. Rules and regulators. Oxford: Clarendon; 1997.

23 Kerrison SH, Pollock AM. Regulating nursing homes: caring for older people in the private sector. British Medical Journal 2001; 323:566–569.

24 Harrington C, Zimmerman D, Karon S, et al. Nursing home staffing levels and its relationship to deficiencies. Journal of Gerontology 2000; 55:278–287. (This paper uses data collected by US federal government on 1.5 m US nursing home residents to demonstrate this relationship.)

25 Hutter BM. Compliance: regulation and environment. Oxford: Oxford University Press; 1997.

26 Hawkins K. Environment and enforcement: regulation and the social definition of pollution. Oxford: Oxford University Press; 1984.

27 Department of Health Press release 2002/0049, 30 January 2002.

28 Department of Health. The care standards tribunal: regulations comprising procedural rules of the Tribunal Consultation Document Care Standards Act 2000. London: Department of Health; 2001.

29 Reichman N. Moving backstage: uncovering the role of compliance practices in shaping regulatory policy. In: Baldwin R, Scott C, Hood C, eds. A reader on regulation. Oxford: Oxford University Press; 1998.

30 Kagan RA. Regulatory enforcement. In: Rosenbloom DH, Schartz RD, eds. Handbook of regulation and administrative law. New York: Marcel Dekker; 1994:383–422.

31 Grabosky P, Braithwaite J. Of gentle manners: enforcement strategies of Australian business regulatory agencies. Oxford: Oxford University Press; 1986.

32 McHarg A. Separation of functions and regulatory agencies: dispute resolution in the privatised utilities. In: Harris M, Partington M, eds. Administrative justice in the 21st century. Oxford: Hart; 1999:125–144.

33 Registered Homes Tribunal decision 306. Online. Available: http://www.doh.gov.uk/rht.

34 Baldwin R. Rules and government. Oxford: Oxford University Press; 1995.

35 Baldwin R, Cave M. Understanding regulation: theory, strategy and practice. Oxford: Oxford University Press; 1999.

36 Ogus A. Regulation: legal form and economic theory. Oxford: Oxford University Press; 1994:116.

37 Justice. A matter of public interest: reforming the law and practice on interventions in public interest cases. London: Justice; 1996.

38 Loux A, Kerrison SH, Pollock AM. Long term nursing: social care or health care? British Medical Journal 2000; 320:5–6.

39 Ayres I, Braithwaite J. Responsive regulation: transcending the deregulation debate. Oxford: Oxford University Press; 1992.

Chapter 6

Disciplinary jurisdiction over the medical and other healthcare professions

Charles Foster

INTRODUCTION

This chapter deals with the disciplinary jurisdiction of the General Medical Council (GMC) over doctors, mentions the issues of appraisal and validation, deals in broad outline with the similar jurisdiction of the Nursing and Midwifery Council (NMC) over nurses, midwives and health visitors, and touches on the still embryonic jurisdiction of the Health Professions Council (HPC), the Council for the Regulation of Healthcare Professionals and the National Clinical Assessment Authority (NCAA).[i]

---

[i] There are many other organisations (such as the National Care Standards Commission and the National Institute for Clinical Excellence) which have some role in maintaining standards in the NHS, but their interest is not primarily in individual healthcare workers and so they are not considered here.

REGULATING THE REGULATORS: THE COUNCIL FOR THE REGULATION OF HEALTHCARE PROFESSIONALS

The NHS Plan published in July 2000 proposed the formation of a UK Council of Health Regulators (http://www.nhs.uk/nhsplan). This would coordinate, but not replace, the activities of the individual healthcare professionals' organisations. It would in effect, regulate the regulators, ensuring that they acted in an appropriately vigilant and mutually consistent way. The Kennedy Report on the Bristol Royal Infirmary Inquiry endorsed this idea, suggesting the title 'Council for the Regulation of Healthcare Professionals' (http://www.bristolinquiry.org.uk/final_report/index.htm). The government agreed, and the Council for the Regulation of Healthcare Professionals sprang into being.[ii] How it will work in practice is not clear, as these are very early days. There is a good deal of cynicism about the Council, the general one being that yet another layer of bureaucracy has been added.

THE NATIONAL CLINICAL ASSESSMENT AUTHORITY

This began work in April 2001.[iii] It is a special health authority, which aims to provide 'a support service to health authorities, primary care trusts and hospital and community trusts who are faced with concerns over the performance of an individual doctor' (http://www.ncaa.nhs.uk). It is an advisory body. When a concern is referred to it, it investigates, assesses, and makes suggestions. It is not a regulator. The employing NHS body remains responsible for resolving the problem.

There is a good deal of potential overlap between the investigations carried out by the NCAA and those carried out by the employing body, the GMC, etc. and it is as yet unclear how these bodies will relate to one another. The NCAA insists that it will liaise closely with bodies like the GMC and the Commission for Health Improvement.

THE DISCIPLINARY JURISDICTION OF THE GMC

The GMC: general

The GMC gets its powers from statute – the Medical Act 1983. The Act provides that: 'The main objective of the General Medical Council in exercising their functions is to protect, promote and maintain the health and safety of the public'.[iv]

[ii] It came into being on 1 April 2003. Sourced from the National Health Service Reform and Health Care Professions Act 2002.
[iii] It was constituted by the National Clinical Assessment Authority (Establishment and Constitution Order) 2000: SI 2000 No. 2961.
[iv] Medical Act 1983, s.1A (inserted by The Medical Act 1983 (Amendment) Order 2002: SI 2002 No. 3135).

The old GMC

The old GMC has been lambasted by the public as being an incestuous closed shop which was so reluctant to criticise doctors that it should no longer be entrusted with the crucial job of regulating the profession. Many doctors have said that it has responded with knee jerk thoughtlessness to media headlines, over-reacting hysterically to allegations that doctors are insufficiently account-able by stringing them up whatever the evidence.

The truth is that the GMC has been terrified of losing the role of regulator. There is justice in the criticism that, particularly as regards matters of pro-fessional conduct, justice to individual doctors has sometimes been sacrificed to the perceived higher purpose of showing the public that the GMC is no soft touch.

The Medical Act has now been radically amended by the Medical Act 1983 (Amendment) Order 2002, and the very scale of the amendments has convinced the GMC that it is not about to be abolished in favour of some quango. That has bred confidence and therefore fairness. The Human Rights Act 1998 (and par-ticularly Article 6 of the European Convention on Human Rights) has forced the various Committees to look hard at their procedure. There are few substantive changes in the procedure. Notably there is a requirement to give reasoned deci-sions, and there is a more obvious separation of the investigative/prosecutorial functions on the one hand and the adjudicatory functions on the other. More significant has been a change in the ethos of adjudication. The Professional Conduct Committee looks warily at possible Article 6 appeals, and more fairly at defendants.

Complaining against doctors is a huge growth industry. In 1995, the Professional Conduct Committee of the GMC sat for 83 days. In 2001, it sat for 479 days. In 1995, the GMC received 1503 complaints: in 2001 it was 4504.[v]

The old GMCs' adjudicatory apparatus consisted of three broad streams which never ran in the same channel – although it was possible sometimes to divert a particular case into one channel from another.[vi]

If a doctor's performance was called into question, without alleged serious professional misconduct, the performance jurisdiction was invoked.[vii] The allegations were examined by a medical and a lay screener. If an assessment was necessary the practitioner was told and asked if he agreed. If he did not agree, the question of whether such an assessment should be carried out was debated before the Assessment Referral Committee.

Assessments were and are long, intrusive, thorough and stressful. They involve detailed scrutiny of a doctor's practice, including observing operations and consultations, tests of clinical competence and knowledge, interviews with

---

[v] Maintaining pace: setting the agenda: General Medical Council, 2002.
[vi] At the time of writing (September 2003) these procedures are still followed, but are referred to in the past tense because they will shortly be redundant.
[vii] See: The General Medical Council (Professional Performance) Rules Order of Council 1997: SI 1997 No. 1529.

professional and lay colleagues and many other strenuous hurdles. Concern following the assessment can lead to the practitioner appearing before the Committee on Professional Performance. The practitioner can be and often is represented at this Committee by counsel or a solicitor. The Committee has to sit with a 'specialist adviser' from the practitioner's specialty who gives advice on medical questions. His opinion is powerful and crucial.

The Committee can suspend or attach conditions to a practitioner's registration. If it was suggested that a doctor's performance was compromised because of his health (usually, in practice, drink, drugs or mental illness), the Health Committee, after obtaining relevant medical reports and hearing submissions, could again suspend or impose conditions.[viii]

The headline-grabbing jurisdiction was the Professional Conduct jurisdiction.[ix] If there was evidence which suggested to a screener and to the Preliminary Proceedings Committee that a practitioner might be guilty of serious professional misconduct,[x] the doctor would find himself in a wood-panelled chamber at the GMC's premises in Hallam Street,[xi] effectively as the defendant in a criminal trial. The press would be there and there would normally be counsel on each side. The standard of proof would be, at least in theory, the criminal standard and a legal assessor would try to keep the Committee from being unlawful.

The Professional Conduct Committee acquired an unfortunate reputation among doctors and lawyers as something of a kangaroo court. It was far more difficult to secure acquittals there than it was in front of a jury, and legal submissions tended to be treated with disdain and distaste – as if they were tricks designed to keep the Committee from its rightful prey.

There was an appeal from the Professional Conduct Committee to the Privy Council. The Privy Council used to be rather passive. It tended to assert, mantra-like, that the Committee was a professional committee with a strong legal rudder and quite capable of assessing evidence in a judicial way and making up its mind about what amounted to serious professional misconduct. Latterly the Privy Council has been more ready to intervene and substitute its own decisions for that of the Committee: that readiness has helped to make for a fairer Committee.

Bridging the performance, health and conduct jurisdictions is the Interim Orders Committee (re-named under the amended Medical Act the Interim Orders Panel).[xii] This began sitting in August 2000. It has the power to interfere

---

[viii] See: The General Medical Council Health Committee (Procedure) Rules Order of Council 1987: SI 1987 No. 2174 amended by SI 1996 No. 1219.
[ix] See: The General Medical Council Preliminary Proceedings Committee and Professional Conduct Committee (Procedure) Rules Order in Council 1988: SI 1988 No. 2255 amended by SI 1989 No. 656, 1990 No. 1587, 1994 No. 2022 and 1996 No. 2125.
[x] A slippery concept, which has systematically evaded definition over the whole course of its life: see, for example, the recent consideration in *GMC* v. *Silver*, unreported, 14 April 2003, Privy Council.
[xi] Or, because the Committees were so hard pressed, in a hotel or rented office accommodation elsewhere in London or, latterly, Manchester.

with a practitioner's registration (by suspension or the imposition of conditions) between the making of the complaint and the eventual adjudication. The test for an order is satisfaction 'that it is necessary for the protection of members of the public or otherwise in the public interest or in the interests of the practitioner'.[xiii]

The Interim Orders Committee has worked well. It has wielded its draconian sanctions efficiently and fairly.

The new GMC

The GMC has been radically changed by the amendments to the Medical Act 1983 mentioned above. It was a big and unwieldy organisation, with 104 Council members. It has now been trimmed to 35 members. The disciplinary procedure has been overhauled. One of the main concerns was the rigidity and artificiality of the old distinctions between health, performance and conduct. In practice, reasons for endangering patients often overlap: sick doctors, for instance, often perform badly and that performance might amount to serious professional misconduct.

The GMC says: 'The key characteristic of the new model is that it is a unitary system which will enable a doctor's fitness to practise to be considered in the round, while nevertheless recognising that different methodologies will be required to deal with different aspects of dysfunctional practice'.[xiv]

There will be two stages in the new Fitness to Practise procedures. The first is the 'Investigation', carried out by the Investigation Committee.[xv] Cases which should not be troubling the GMC can still be closed by the Registrar and his staff: anything not falling into that class is processed by the investigation machinery. What amounts to appropriate investigation will vary hugely from case to case.

The basic question which the Committee must answer is whether there is a realistic prospect of establishing that the doctor's fitness to practise is impaired to a degree justifying action on his registration (Medical Act 1983, s.35D(2)). A doctor's fitness to practise shall be regarded as 'impaired' for these purposes, by reason only of: '(a) misconduct (b) deficient professional performance (c) a conviction or caution in the British Islands for a criminal offence or a conviction elsewhere for an offence which, if committed in England and Wales, would constitute a criminal offence (d) adverse physical or mental health or (e) a determination by a body in the United Kingdom responsible under any enactment for the regulation of a health or social care profession to the effect

---

[xii] See: The General Medical Council (Interim Orders Committee) (Procedure) Rules Order of Council 2000: SI 2000 No. 2053.

[xiii] The General Medical Council (Interim Orders Committee) (Procedure) Rules Order of Council 2000: SI 2000 No. 2053 Article 11(9).

[xiv] Review of Fitness to Practise: The New Model. General Medical Council, November 2002. Online. Available: http://www.gmc-uk.org/about/reform/ftpmodel_rev.htm

[xv] The functions of the Investigation Committee are set out in s.35C of the Medical Act 1983.

that his fitness to practise as a member of that profession is impaired, or a determination by a regulatory body elsewhere to the same effect'.[xvi] Professional performance is specifically stated to include competence (Medical Act 1983, s.55). If there is such a prospect, the complaint moves on to the next stage, 'Adjudication'. If there is no such prospect, two outcomes are possible. The first is that no action is taken by the GMC, although there might be referral to an NHS or other local compliance or disciplinary body. If, however, it is considered that in the interests of maintaining good professional standards and public confidence in the profession some formal response is necessary, the Investigation Committee has the power to issue a warning to a doctor if either there has been a significant departure from good medical practice, or a GMC performance assessment has indicated cause for concern about the doctor's performance, considered as a whole. A doctor has a right to an oral hearing before a warning is issued. A warning will not normally be disclosed to anyone other than the doctor, his employer and any complainant and will remain on the doctor's file for the purposes of appraisal and revalidation for 5 years.

If the matter does go on to the Adjudication stage, it passes into the hands of a Fitness to Practise Panel.[xvii] Although the idea is to have a holistic approach, so that fitness to practise generally is considered, there are still separate streams for conduct, conviction, health and performance. The Committee can only take action if the appropriate process has been followed for the type of case the Committee ultimately considers the one in question to be. For example, the Committee could not start a case as a conduct case, conclude *en route* that the doctor's performance was really the issue and act on a finding of deficient performance, without ordering the usual performance assessment.

The procedure will be very similar to that followed in old proceedings, before the Professional Conduct Committee. In particular, the standard of proof remains the criminal standard. This has been controversial. There was vocal support for the civil standard throughout and for a sliding standard to be applied – 'criminal', if essentially criminal allegations were being made, sliding down to the 'balance of probabilities', where the allegations did not contain allegations of impropriety.

Where the Committee finds that a practitioner's fitness to practise is impaired, it can erase his name from the register (except where the allegations are in relation to health), suspend for not more than 1 year, or impose conditions for not more than 3 years (Medical Act 1983, s.35D(2)). If it finds that fitness to practise is not impaired, it can nevertheless 'give him a warning regarding his future conduct or performance'.[xviii]

[xvi] Medical Act 1983, s.35C(2). Section 35C(3) gives explicit extraterritorial effect and provides that the Committee can consider allegations relating to a time when the doctor was not registered with the GMC.
[xvii] The functions of the Fitness to Practise Panel are set out in 35D of the Medical Act 1983.
[xviii] Medical Act 1983, s.35D(3). There is no appeal against such a warning.

Appeals are to the High Court. There is no requirement for permission to appeal and no requirement that the appeal is on a question of law alone. The Court's powers are wide: it can dismiss the appeal, allow it and quash the Committee's decision, substitute any other decision which the Committee could have made, or remit for redetermination (Medical Act 1983, s.40).

No commencement date for most of these provisions has yet been announced.[xix] The word on the medical street suggests some time in 2004.

Registration, revalidation and appraisal

To practise medicine in the UK, a doctor has to be registered with the GMC. By 1 January 2005, it will not be enough merely to be registered: it will be necessary to be licensed to practise. The first licences will be given to all doctors who are on the GMC's register by the end of 2004. Licences will have to be renewed every 5 years. To renew a licence it will be necessary for a doctor to show that he conducts his practice in accordance with the principles in the GMC's bible *Good Medical Practice*.[1] The process of demonstrating compliance and obtaining a licence is called revalidation.[xx]

There is no set way in which doctors must demonstrate compliance, but there are broadly two main ways. The first, which the vast majority of doctors will use, is the 'Appraisal' route. This applies to doctors who work within a 'managed environment' and who have participated in an annual appraisal system. There are or will be appraisal schemes to cover all doctors with NHS contracts, including academics and managers and the GMC states that 'doctors included on General Medical Services lists, Personal Medical Services contracts and supplementary lists held by Primary Care Organisations can consider themselves as working within a managed environment'[xxi] – an observation which will be greeted by many patients with surprised relief. The second option is the 'Independent' route. This will be used by many outside the NHS (although doctors working in hospitals, which are members of the Independent Healthcare Association, are likely to find that they are in an endorsed 'managed environment'). Followers of this route will be required to keep self-audit records of the type now required in the NHS and demonstrate that they have clocked enough hours in continuing medical education.

For most doctors in the NHS, this is not going to make a lot of difference. The initiative is really a public relations exercise. It is unlikely to do more than the existing complaint, performance and conduct procedures, but it will be helpful for the public: they will gain more confidence in the profession.

There is a link between the revalidation/appraisal procedures and the performance procedures: inadequate evidence to ensure revalidation is likely to lead to a performance assessment.

[xix] Some provisions, including those relating to the composition of the GMC, have been in force since 17 December 2002.

[xx] The details are summarised and discussed at http://www.gmc-uk.org/revalidation

[xxi] The details are summarised and discussed at http://www.gmc-uk.org/revalidation

THE DISCIPLINARY JURISDICTION OF THE NMC

The NMC: general

The NMC came into being on 1 April 2002, taking over the function of the United Kingdom Central Council for Nursing, Midwifery and Health Visiting (UKCC).[xxii] It was formally created by the Nursing and Midwifery Order 2001 (SI 2002 No. 253). The Order provides that: 'The principal functions of the Council shall be to establish from time to time standards of education, training, conduct and performance for nurses and midwives and to ensure the maintenance of those standards' (Article 3(2)).

Investigation and adjudication of complaints

Complaints against registered nurses, midwives and health visitors have risen significantly over recent years. In 1996–1997 the UKCC received 893 complaints: in 2000–2001 there were 1240. The UKCC's Preliminary Proceedings Committee considered 1627 cases in 2000–2001, referring 221 to the Professional Conduct Committee.[2]

Just as for the GMC, the NMC's fitness to practise procedures have been radically changed by legislation. Articles 21 to 36 of the Nursing and Midwifery Order lay down a comprehensive system for assessing fitness to practise. There is an Investigating Committee (Article 26), a Conduct and Competence Committee (Article 27), a Health Committee (Article 28) and provision for interim orders (Article 31). Subject to consultation, the Conduct and Competence Committee has agreed to work to the following definition of 'lack of competence': 'A lack of knowledge, skill or judgement, which may be accompanied by a negative attitude. This is of such a nature that the nurse, midwife or health visitor is unfit to practise and that such concerns having been drawn to the attention of the practitioner, he or she has either undergone training and supervision but has failed to make the required improvement to practice, or has refused to undergo further training or supervision'.[3] The orders the Health and Conduct and Competence Committees may make are to take no action, to strike the practitioner off the register, to suspend registration for a maximum of 1 year, to impose conditions for up to 3 years, or to caution the practitioner and note the caution on the register for not less than one and not more than 5 years (Article 29(5)). Striking off is not an option for lack of competence or health unless the practitioner has been under conditions or suspended continuously for at least 2 years immediately before the order (Article 29(6)). Procedure within these Committees is similar to the procedure at the GMC. There is an appeal to the High Court (Article 38). Similar comments apply as to appeals from the GMC's procedures.

[xxii] Further details of its function and procedures are available from its website at: http://www.nmc-uk.org

The NMC's system is therefore something of a hybrid of the old and new GMC system – putting investigation of all complaints under one administrative roof, combining jurisdiction over conduct and competence at the adjudication stage, but maintaining a distinct health committee.

THE DISCIPLINARY JURISDICTION OF THE HPC

The HPC: general

The HPC replaces the old Council for Professions Supplementary to Medicine. It was set up by the Health Professions Order 2001 (http://www.hpc-uk.org). It regulates arts, music and drama therapists, chiropodists, podiatrists, clinical scientists, dieticians, medical laboratory technicians, occupational therapists, orthoptists, prosthetists, orthotists, paramedics, physiotherapists, radiographers, speech and language therapists and operating department practitioners.

Investigation and adjudication of complaints

The Health Professions Order 2001 contains detailed provision for the investigation and adjudication of complaints (Articles 21–36). They are practically identical to those of the NMC and there is similarly an appeal to the High Court. It has yet to be seen how these procedures will work in practice.

CONCLUSION

For a time, it seemed that self-regulation of the healthcare professions was in jeopardy. The danger now seems to have passed. New legislation has made (or will make) the disciplinary procedures more flexible, less in thrall to the artificial distinctions between professional misconduct, professional performance and health which characterised the old system, and better able to do the job of protecting the public.

References

1 GMC. Good Medical Practice. GMC; September 2001.
2 UKCC. Professional Conduct Annual Report, 2000–2001. London: UKCC; November 2001.
3 NMC News, April 2003:6.

Chapter **7**

The implications of the Human Rights Act 1998 – prioritising consent

Elizabeth Wicks

INTRODUCTION – A HUMAN RIGHTS AGE

We live in a human rights age. Irrespective of arguments as to the potential benefits of this (to both individual autonomy and society as a whole), it is an unavoidable fact that English law now requires respect for the fundamental civil and political rights of individuals. And, contrary to some paternalistic approaches, medical patients are, first and foremost, individuals entitled to respect for their rights. Of prime importance within a doctor–patient context is the patient's right to be free of degrading treatment and to have respect paid to his or her right to a private life (incorporating a right to physical integrity). In short, human rights norms embody the idea of self-determination – as to medical treatment, as well as to other choices in life.

The Human Rights Act 1998 (HRA) gives further effect in English law to the fundamental rights and freedoms contained in the European Convention on Human Rights (ECHR), to which the UK has been a party for over half a century. The HRA creates no new rights and it falls short of the stringent enforcement methods favoured by many public law commentators. The UK Parliament remains supreme (perhaps 'sovereign', whatever that ambiguous term may mean) and retains authority to violate the rights of its citizens (albeit only if done in express terms). But, for all its limitations and lack of radicalism, the HRA transforms the constitutional climate in the UK. It does this at a political and presentational level, and also by empowering the British judiciary to be proactive in upholding individual rights. That the courts have accepted this opportunity is evident in many areas of law, not least medical law. What is equally apparent is that the potential implications of the courts doing so have not yet been realised by all the medical profession.

This chapter seeks to investigate the implications of the HRA for the medical and legal professions' respective approaches to the choices of patients. It identifies three changes wrought by the HRA: a change in the form in which judges adjudicate on these matters; a change in the substance of English law on consent; and a change in the consequence of ignoring this recent prioritisation of consent. The medical profession will ignore these changes at their peril.

THE RIGHTS-BASED APPROACH TO MEDICAL LAW: A CHANGE IN FORM?

Arguably, the most obvious change wrought by the HRA to medical law cases is one of form rather than substance. The courts have discovered, adopted (and adapted) a rights-based approach to medico-legal issues. Many may feel that this is a long overdue development. Traditionally, the relevant domestic law has been framed in terms of doctors' duties.[i] For example, a claim of medical negligence will depend upon a doctor falling below a standard of care determined by professional colleagues.[ii] This body of medical opinion is also determinative of the information released to patients concerning the risks of treatment (*Sidaway* v. *Board of Governors of the Bethlam Royal Hospital* [1985] 1 All ER 643) and of the treatment of an incompetent patient in his or her best interests.[iii] The rights of the patient were rarely acknowledged, let alone protected by courts pre-HRA. But this must now change.[iv] The enactment of the

---

[i] This approach led to a tendency for the courts to treat the medical profession 'with excessive deference'. Lord Woolf has recognised that this has its potential dangers: 'it is unwise to place any profession or other body providing services to the public on a pedestal where their actions cannot be subject to close scrutiny'. (Lord Woolf, 'Are the Courts Excessively Deferential to the Medical Profession?' Medical Law Review 2001; 9:1–15.)

[ii] The infamous Bolam test has long stalked the body of negligence. First expressed in *Bolam* v. *Friern Hospital Management Committee* [1957] 1 WLR 583, the test was subsequently adopted by the House of Lords in *Whitehouse* v. *Jordan* [1981] 1 All ER 267 and *Maynard* v. *West Midlands RHA* [1985] 1 All ER 635. The test still determines the standard of care in negligence although a gloss was placed upon it in *Bolitho* v. *City and Hackney Health Authority* [1998] AC 232.

[iii] *Re F (Mental Patient: Sterilisation)* [1990] 2 AC 1, although more recent cases (e.g. *Re S (Adult Patient: Sterilisation)* [2000] 3 WLR 1288) have acknowledged that the Bolam test must be supplemented by wider ethical, social and moral considerations (which are not necessarily best determined by doctors).

[iv] Lord Irvine of Lairg, the former Lord Chancellor, noted a 'movement towards recognition of circumstances in which practices considered appropriate by a body of doctors may not always be the benchmark by which their actions may be judged'. (Lord Irvine of Lairg. The patient, the doctor, their lawyers and the judge: rights and duties. Medical Law Review 1999; 7:255–268.)

HRA has forced a recognition that Kennedy and Grubb were correct to claim medical law as a 'subset of human rights law'.[1] The guiding philosophy of decisions concerning medical treatment must now be the rights of the patient, rather than the duties of the doctor. The HRA provides a starting point, a legal framework and a guiding light. And its most noticeable impact is in encouraging a new language of rights.

A useful indication of the transformation in judicial thinking is provided by a comparison of the courts' approach in the pre-HRA case of *Re T* (*a minor*) (*wardship: medical treatment*) [1997] 1 All ER 906, and the conjoined twins case of *Re A* (*children*) (*conjoined twins: surgical separation*) [2000] 4 All ER 961, decided only days before the HRA came into force. In *Re T*, a mother refused to give consent for her child to undergo a liver transplant, essential if he was to survive beyond 2½ years of age, because she did not want him to be subjected to invasive surgery. The Court of Appeal overturned the first instance decision to authorise the operation against the mother's wishes. The Court of Appeal judges were adamant that the welfare of the child (a key family law principle) was paramount. This principle enabled the court to argue that '[t]he welfare of this child depends upon his mother' (*Re T* (*a minor*) (*wardship: medical treatment*) [1997] 1 All ER 915) and that, therefore, an operation against her express wishes would be unproductive: 'the best interests of this child require that his future treatment should be left in the hands of his devoted parents' (*Re T* (*a minor*) (*wardship: medical treatment*) [1997] 1 All ER 916). This beneficence, or welfare, approach is evident in many important English medical cases,[v] often at the expense of individual autonomy, and can be distinguished from a rights-based approach. Not once in the Court of Appeal's judgment in *Re T* is there acknowledgement of the implications of the decision for T's right to life. Indeed, Waite LJ expressly stated that: 'It is not an occasion – even in an age preoccupied with "rights" – to talk of the rights of the child, or the rights of a parent, or the rights of the court' (*Re T* (*a minor*) (*wardship: medical treatment*) [1997] 1 All ER 916). If this were not such an occasion, one may legitimately wonder when such an occasion would arise. In 1996, when this case was decided, the UK was bound at international law to the ECHR, including Article 2's fundamental protection of a right to life. In addition, as Brooke LJ recognised in the later case of *Re A*: 'the fundamental importance of the right to protection of life' was already 'ingrained in the English common law' (*Re A* (*children*) (*conjoined twins: surgical separation*) [2000] 4 All ER 1050). There was no excuse, therefore, for a failure to recognise that T had a right to life which, although not absolute, required specific and reasoned justification for its departure.

If *Re T* avoided the use of a language of rights, *Re A* embraced it. Although the HRA was 10 days away from coming into force, the Court of Appeal

---

[v] See, for example, *Re T* (*Adult: Refusal of Medical Treatment*) [1992] 4 All ER 649; *Re S* (*Adult: Refusal of Medical Treatment*) [1992] 4 All ER 671; and *Re F* (*Mental Patient: Sterilisation*) [1990] 2 AC 1.

worked within the ECHR's framework. Hence, the key issue for the judges was how to balance two conflicting rights to life.[vi] In this unique factual situation, the language of rights was ultimately unhelpful. The right of one of the twins would have to be favoured over the other's, thus negating the equality inherent in the right to life. Ward LJ was at pains to point out, however, that it was the 'worthwhileness of treatment' which was being compared, rather than the respective value of each twin's life: 'The universality of the right to life demands that the right to life be treated as equal. The intrinsic value of their human life is equal. So the right of each goes into the scales and the scales remain in balance' (*Re A (children) (conjoined twins: surgical separation)* [2000] 4 All ER 1050). This explicit recognition that each twin had a right to life is a welcome departure from the Court of Appeal's approach in the earlier case of *Re T*. And, although it was claimed in respect of the HRA that 'in this case its effect is to confirm, and not to alter, pre-existing law' (at 1068), it is unlikely that such an emphasis upon the rights and interests of the twins would have been regarded as necessary without the imminent incorporation of the ECHR. The form in which the judgment was presented – the language used – has been transformed.

This can be seen even more clearly in another recent landmark case, that of Dianne Pretty (*R (on the application of Pretty)* v. *DPP* [2002] 1 All ER 1; *Dianne Pretty* v. *United Kingdom* [2002] 35 EHRR 1). Here, the claimant, in seeking an undertaking that her husband would not be prosecuted for assisting her to commit suicide, relied upon various rights under the Convention. For example, she claimed that a right to die was inherent in a right to life and that her right to respect for a private life entailed a right to choose the manner and time of her own death. The House of Lords was required to answer each point of her claim in some detail, hence the judgment is almost entirely comprised of rights-based analysis. The fact that Pretty was unsuccessful in claiming her 'right to die' does not detract from the transformation in medical law post-HRA, of which this case is indicative. Indeed, without the HRA, Pretty would have had no possible cause of action. The case illustrates, therefore, that the changes in the medico-legal landscape have been significant in terms of the form of post-HRA judgments. But the most significant implication of the HRA has yet to be discussed. This focuses on a change in substance – the prioritisation of consent.

PRIORITISING CONSENT: A CHANGE IN SUBSTANCE?

Consent has always formed an essential part of English law. The general principle was propounded in the 1992 case of *Re T (Adult: Refusal of Medical Treatment)* [1992] 4 All ER 649. The Court of Appeal emphasised that an adult

---

[vi]The weaker twin would inevitably die as a result of the separation but, without it, both twins would survive for only a few months. The parents were opposed to the operation, preferring to allow nature to run its course.

of sound mind has the right to give or refuse consent to medical treatment. The reasons for a refusal of consent are, it was held, irrelevant. If a competent adult says no, the treatment cannot be imposed, regardless of the doctor's opinions as to the best interests and clinical needs of the patient and regardless of the likely consequences of the refusal. Even a refusal of treatment, which will certainly lead to death must be respected, see *Re B* (*Adult: Refusal of Medical Treatment*) [2002] 2 All ER 449. These various elements of the principle of consent were effectively expressed by Lord Donaldson of Lymington MR:

> 'An adult patient who, like Miss T, suffers from no mental incapacity has an absolute right to choose whether to consent to medical treatment, to refuse it or to choose one rather than another of the treatments being offered … This right of choice is not limited to decisions which others might regard as sensible. It exists notwithstanding that the reasons for making the choice are rational, irrational, unknown or even non-existent' (*Re T* (*Adult: Refusal of Medical Treatment*) [1992] 4 All ER 650–653).

The general principle, then, is clear. It enshrines autonomy into English law. The ambiguity arises on the borderline of competence.

The crucial proviso inherent within the general need for consent to medical treatment is that the patient must be mentally competent to make a choice as regards treatment. In practice, this requirement has not merely protected the welfare of the mentally ill or unconscious patient, but has also excluded temporarily distressed, confused or irrational patients from the ambit of the consent principle. This has led to a worrying dichotomy in English medical law. On the one hand, English law has shown an impressive commitment to the general need for consent. Higher courts, in landmark cases, have eloquently declared the fundamental nature of a patient's autonomy. On the other hand, it cannot be denied that English law has revealed an unfortunate tendency to undermine the principle in practice by demonstrating an excessive willingness to declare non-consenting patients to be incompetent. The evidence suggests that courts have, on occasion, upheld the medical profession's practice of regarding a refusal of consent to act as an indicator of a lack of competence. If a patient says 'no' to treatment which is objectively in his or her best interests – which, indeed, may be necessary to save the patient's life – this could be regarded by both the legal and medical profession as evidence that the patient is irrational and unable to make a responsible choice regarding treatment. But, as was emphasised in *Re T* (and numerous other cases), the patient's choice need not be rational or responsible. It is a right to choose, not a right to make the objectively correct choice.

The dilemma facing the medical profession in this context relates to the ethical duties upon doctors as to treatment of their patients. It must be acknowledged that doctors do not impose non-consensual treatment on a patient in a thoughtless or arbitrary manner. If they do impose such treatment, they do so because saving lives is the epitome of their professional duty. Since the Hippocratic oath first declared that a doctor should act 'for the good' of his patient and 'never do harm', a paternalistic approach has dominated the profession. And so it should, for beneficence is at the core of providing health care. But such a duty of care must never overwhelm the rights of the patient. As the Lord Chancellor has noted, the HRA introduces a potential conflict here: 'if incorporation of the European Convention on Human Rights encourages the courts to focus more on the patients' rights, this may prove not entirely compatible with what doctors have traditionally seen as their duties'.[2] If rights and duties conflict, the rights of the patient should take priority, but it must be acknowledged that such reconciliation is not always easy to achieve.

A good example of a perceived conflict between a patient's rights and a doctor's duty is provided by the 1998 case of *St George's Healthcare NHS Trust v. S* [1998] 3 All ER 673. A woman who was 36 weeks pregnant was diagnosed with pre-eclampsia. She was advised that she needed to be admitted to hospital for an induced delivery, but she refused and insisted on a natural birth. Without this induced delivery, both her life and the life of her unborn child were in danger. What were her doctors to do? The choice of the woman's medical carers was, astonishingly, to admit her to a mental hospital for assessment under Section 2 of the Mental Health Act 1983 and apply *ex parte* to the courts for a declaration dispensing with the need for her to consent to treatment. Hogg J granted the declaration. The woman was duly subjected to a caesarean section delivery against her will. Two days later her compulsory detention under the Mental Health Act was terminated. At no time was any treatment for a mental disorder prescribed, nor was there any medical evidence for such a disorder (other than a few comments that she was probably depressed). The case was later appealed and, in a prime example of the dichotomy between theory and practice (and between higher courts and emergency hearings), the Court of Appeal made clear that both the doctors and the court had chosen to resolve this dilemma in an erroneous way. At no point in the court hearing was the issue of the woman's competence considered and yet, if she was competent (and no evidence was provided that she was not), she had the right to refuse consent. Judge LJ expressed this point extremely clearly in the Court of Appeal when he queried, 'how can a forced invasion of a competent adult's body against her will even for the most laudable of motives (the preservation of life) be ordered without irremediably damaging the principle of self-determination?' (*St George's Healthcare NHS Trust v. S* [1998] 3 All ER 688.) He went on to say that 'the autonomy of each individual requires continuing protection even, perhaps particularly, when the motive for interfering with it is readily understandable, and indeed to many would appear commendable' (*St George's Healthcare NHS Trust v. S* [1998] 3 All ER 688). This, of course, is the dilemma facing both the medical profession and the judiciary in such situations: treating without consent appears 'commendable' and the right thing to do, because it will save life, but the cost in human rights terms is simply too high. It is vital that neither English law nor medical practice continues to implement this dangerous practice of using the choice made as evidence of the ability to choose. Not only is this practice unethical but now, due to the HRA, there is a strong argument that it is unlawful.

Consent in the Convention

The principle of autonomy is inherent in the civil and political rights and free-doms protected in the ECHR. It underlies the Convention without ever being expressly identified. In fact, if one guiding principle were to be sought from the text of the Convention it would, no doubt, be the principle of democracy. The ECHR sought to preserve a democratic peace within Western Europe at a time of totalitarian threat. The Council of Europe identified the international protection of civil and political rights and freedoms as the most effective means of doing this and included some permissible limitations of rights when 'necessary in a democratic society' in order to achieve a legitimate societal aim. However, at the core of the rights and freedoms is individual autonomy. In summary form, this is the right to choose – the right to choose how to live, to choose when and how to express oneself, to choose a religion (or not), to choose whether to permit encroachments into one's own physical integrity or not. Included within this general right to choose is a right to choose or reject medical treatment. It is an essential element in a philosophy based upon autonomy. It prioritises consent as the fundamental principle in providing quality health care.

The applicability of the Convention rights to consent issues in medical care does not rest solely upon this general ethos of the Convention, however. The ability to make choices in the intimate area of medical treatment is implicitly referred to in the specific Articles of the Convention. Article 3, for example, prohibits (*inter alia*) the imposition of degrading treatment. The European Commission of Human Rights has previously held that 'medical treatment of an experimental character and without the consent of the person involved may under certain circumstances be regarded as prohibited by Article 3' (*X v. Denmark* [1983] 32 DR 282 at 283). At the other extreme, 'a measure which is a therapeutic necessity cannot be regarded as inhuman or degrading' but the European Court of Human Rights made clear in the *Herczegfalvy* case that such 'medical necessity' must be proven ((1992) Series A, No. 244). Thus, under Article 3, imposing treatment without consent may under certain circumstances be regarded as degrading, although therapeutic necessity, if proven, will usually provide a sufficient excuse. This may not be sufficient, however, under Article 8 where the right to respect for a private life incorpor-ates a right to physical integrity of the person (*X & Y v. Netherlands* [1986] 8 EHRR 235 at para. 22). The Commission has stated that a 'compulsory med-ical intervention' must be considered an interference with Article 8, although this is not an absolute right and, in the case in question, the compulsory blood test to determine paternity was justified as necessary in a democratic society to protect the rights of others. Article 8 protects the freedom to make one's own choices and so non-consensual treatment on a competent patient would unarguably fall foul of this provision. Indeed, in the recent *Pretty* case, the European Court of Human Rights indicated a willingness to accept the applic-ability of Article 8 to life and death decisions (*Dianne Pretty v. United Kingdom* [2002] 35 EHRR 1). In addition, a refusal to consent to treatment on religious grounds may raise an argument under Article 9's freedom to manifest a religion or belief. In short, then, the HRA incorporates the idea of autonomy and free choice to the UK, both through its presence in the overall ethos of the Convention and its role in underlying many specific rights.[vii] What has been the impact of the incorporation of such ideas?

The dire need for the incorporation of such ideas from the ECHR (and English common law) into medical practice is illustrated by the recent case of *Re B (Adult: Refusal of Medical Treatment)* [2002] 2 All ER 449. This case is illuminating, not only because it clarifies the importance of consent in English law post-HRA (and, arguably, pre-HRA), but also because it highlights the apparent lack of awareness of this fact amongst some members of the medical profession. Ms B was tetraplegic and sustained by means of artificial ventilation. She was fully conscious and, crucially, mentally competent.[viii] Despite this, her repeated requests for artificial ventilation to cease were refused, forcing her to take legal action to assert this established right to refuse treatment. See *Re T (Adult: Refusal of Medical Treatment)* [1992] 4 All ER 649 and *Re C (Adult: Refusal of Treatment)* [1994] 1 All ER 819. The case was not, as the press would have had us believe, about the right to die. It was not comparable to the Dianne Pretty case. It was instead concerned with the right to refuse consent to medical treatment. In the absence of Ms B's consent, continuing to ventilate her amounted to an unlawful assault upon her person – an infringement of her physical integrity – for which she was awarded damages against the hospital trust. Having determined, following psychiatric evidence, that Ms B was competent to consent or refuse consent to treatment, the Court of Appeal was correct to emphasise that the choice of whether to accept treatment was, unambiguously, Ms B's to make. In law, this was never in doubt but Butler-Sloss LJ recognised that there exist practical difficulties in applying the law in this area:

> 'The general law on mental capacity is, in my judgement, clear and easily to be understood by lawyers. Its application to individual cases in the context of a general practitioner's surgery, a hospital ward and especially in an intensive care unit is infinitely more difficult to achieve' (*Re B (Adult: Refusal of Medical Treatment)* [2002] 2 All ER 449).

In other words, it is one thing for lawyers to frame general rules, but quite another for doctors to apply them in clinical situations. As undoubtedly true as this is, it cannot serve to excuse a systematic departure from the law in this context. The Court of Appeal specifically referred to the particular difficulty in accepting a refusal of treatment in an ICU context. Butler-Sloss LJ said that in an ICU, the medical and nursing team are 'dedicated to saving and preserving life' and that a refusal of consent was 'outside their experience' (*Re B (Adult:*

[vii] See: Wicks E. The right to refuse medical treatment under the European Convention on Human Rights. Medical Law Review 2001; 9:17, for more detailed analysis of the applicability of specific rights to this issue.
[viii] This fact was acknowledged by the hospital's own psychiatrists.

Refusal of Medical Treatment) [2002] 2 All ER 473). This is, then, an area where urgent improvements are required in relation to an appreciation by the medical profession of the relevant legal norms.

As has previously been noted, the danger inherent in assessing capacity is that undue attention will be paid to the decision made, rather than to the capacity to make it. This is, arguably, what occurred in practice in the case of Ms B and thus prevented her choice being given effect for so long. Butler-Sloss LJ gave clear guidance on this issue for the future:

> 'It is most important that those considering the issue should not confuse the question of mental capacity with the nature of the decision made by the patient, however grave the consequences. The view of the patient may reflect a difference in values rather than an absence of competence and the assessment of capacity should be approached with this firmly in mind' (*Re B* (*Adult: Refusal of Medical Treatment*) [2002] 2 All ER 474).

This is an important lesson that must be learnt by the entire medical profession. However much one may disagree with a refusal of treatment, there is no legal authority to treat a competent adult without his consent. Nor should there be. To treat without consent is to commit an unlawful assault. English law has always been clear on this point, but rarely has a case so starkly demonstrated the implications of this principle. Ms B's case was decided without explicit reference to the Human Rights Act – such reference was unnecessary – but no other outcome would have been compatible with the HRA or the ethos behind the Convention. This point is significant and the somewhat complacent view of Grubb on the pre-existing common law is misplaced:

> 'In an era when the Human Rights Act 1998 and the European Convention on Human Rights are so often relied upon to found a legal right, in this instance the common law provided the right and the legal solution. Indeed, the common law is probably more robust in its recognition of a competent patient's right to refuse life-sustaining medical treatment than is the ECHR.'[3]

This view, surely, overstates the protection offered by the common law. It was certainly not 'robust' in *Re S* (*Adult: Refusal of Medical Treatment*) [1992] 4 All ER 671 (in which a competent adult was unable to validly refuse an emergency caesarean section operation on religious grounds) nor in *Re T* (*Adult: Refusal of Medical Treatment*) [1992] 4 All ER 649 (in which a woman suffering from no mental disorder was regarded as incompetent to refuse a blood transfusion, due to the 'undue influence' exerted by her mother). But, more significantly, even if English common law has proved more robust in its protection of autonomy in recent cases (such as *Re B*), medical practice remains undeterred in its paternalistic approach to life and death issues. Hence, Ms B's protestations against artificial ventilation went unheeded and another patient, Miss S, discussed above, was admitted to a mental hospital for refusing a caesarean section operation (*St George's Healthcare NHS Trust* v. *S* [1998] 3 All ER 673). It is in changing the preconceptions of medical practice that the HRA may prove most valuable, for the spectre of illegality now surfaces in relation to violations of self-determination of medical treatment.

ILLEGALITY: A CHANGE IN CONSEQUENCE?

The concept of self-determination, and its applicability within the medical context, has long been established within the UK. In the abstract, there is no doubt that the common law enshrines principles of self-determination and consent (as well as the opposing principles of beneficence and sanctity of life). The difference post-HRA is that a failure to respect such ideas by a public authority (within the context of the Convention rights) is an unlawful act (s.6(1) HRA). An NHS trust will be defined under the HRA as a public authority and so, significantly, will a court and, therefore, a degree of 'horizontal effect' between individual parties before a court is arguable.[ix] If the principle of self-determination is infringed within the context of the Convention rights – e.g. under Article 8's right to respect for private life or Article 3's prohibition of degrading treatment or Article 9's freedom to manifest a religion or belief – the public authority responsible for the infringement, or even, arguably, the private body or individual (via horizontal effect), will have committed an unlawful act and appropriate remedies will be available.[x] Furthermore, the domestic courts must now ensure – and have indeed done so – that the common law develops in a manner consistent with the underlying values of the ECHR. For example, *Re A*, *Re B* and *Pretty* all ensure compliance with the Convention, whether expressly or implicitly.

The existence of the Convention rights within enforceable domestic law will not, of course, always guarantee the success of a rights-based argument. The Convention itself promotes a delicate balance between individual freedom and wider societal interests. For example, the rights of others may justify limitations to an individual's right to respect for private life, as may the protection of health and morals (Article 8(2) ECHR). These justifiable limitations are a consequence of the core role played by 'democratic society' within the Convention. In addition, the HRA is not without its limitations as to enforceability. An Act of Parliament could never be struck down under the HRA and a public authority, which violates a Convention right merely by giving effect to another Act of Parliament, has a defence against an allegation of

---

[ix]On the surface, the HRA only gives vertical effect to the Convention rights – i.e. they are only enforceable against the state or public bodies, not between private bodies or individuals. But, under Section 6(3), courts and tribunals are expressly declared to be 'public authorities'. Some commentators have used this fact to argue that indirect horizontal effect is created by the HRA – i.e. even in a case between two private individuals, the court must reach a decision that conforms with the Convention rights or else it will have acted unlawfully. For differing views on this academic argument, see Buxton R. The Human Rights Act and Private Law (2000) 116 LQR 48 and HWR Wade, 'Horizons of Horizontality' (2000) 116 LQR 217.

[x]'Just and appropriate' (but existing) remedies are available under Section 8 HRA.

unlawfulness (s.6(2) HRA). Nevertheless, the rights-based arguments are now, for the first time, a legal ground for judicial review of public authorities, rather than merely a moral influence. The perceived rights of patients will not always be compatible with existing medical paternalism, nor with legal acquiescence in it. Those providing medical care must be increasingly vigilant to ensure that paternalistic tendencies do not lead them into the territory of illegality. Judges must be equally vigilant that deference to the medical profession does not also lead them to stray onto this territory. The legal and medical landscape is changing.

CONCLUSION

The Human Rights Act 1998 is a timely addition to English public law. It acknowledges (in a domestic, enforceable and unambiguous manner) the rights to which we are all entitled under international human rights treaties and, arguably, the common law constitution. Indeed, the changes wrought by the HRA are all the more surprising when it is appreciated that individual rights are not a new phenomenon in the UK. Fundamental rights have always been inherent in the British democratic constitution.[xi] However, within this uncodified, common law (and, some would argue, descriptive[xii]) constitution, the existence of fundamental rights has not always been properly recognised by the courts. It has taken the export of these rights to Europe (via the ECHR) and back again (via the HRA) for the courts finally to accept their practical implications within the British constitution. Only in the age of the Human Rights Act has the British judiciary been forced to uphold human rights at the threat of illegality. Within a medical context, the implications of this overdue recognition are wide ranging and significant. There can be no doubt that pre-existing English law has failed, on occasion, to uphold the rights of patients, particularly in the sense of self-determination on issues of treatment. The need for consent was acknowledged (indeed, rhapsodised) by the courts but proved to be ineffective all too often in the most problematic of cases. The underlying reason for this failure of English law always to uphold patient autonomy was the judiciary's deference to the medical profession. Emphasis upon the ethical duties and professional standards of doctors inevitably undermined consideration of the rights of patients. The HRA acts as a reminder that

---

[xi] The existence of fundamental common law rights can be traced back to the seventeenth century. See, for example, the Coke doctrine exemplified in Dr Bonham's Case (1610) 8 Co Rep 107a. More recently, the idea has been rediscovered following a period of abeyance (influenced by the Diceyian tradition). Sir John Laws has been particularly influential on this point, both judicially (*Thoburn* v. *Sunderland City Council* [2002] 4 All ER 156, especially paras 62–64) and in his extra-judicial writings (Law and Democracy. PL 1995; 72–93).

[xii] The term 'descriptive' is used here in contrast to a 'prescriptive' constitution. In other words, many commentators (but not the author) deny the British constitution the higher law status common to all other so-called constitutions.

this is unacceptable within a democratic society adhering to the rule of law. The Act encourages the use of a framework (and language) of rights when courts are adjudicating on medico-legal issues; it ensures that patient autonomy, in terms of the need for consent, is prioritised; and it provides a means by which this principle can be effectively enforced. Legal regulation of healthcare quality has a new, and potentially more effective, dimension.

References

1 Kennedy I, Grubb A. Medical law: text and materials, 3rd edn. London: Butterworths; 2000:3.
2 Lord Irvine of Lairg. The patient, the doctor, their lawyers and the judge: rights and duties. Medical Law Review 1999; 7:255–268.
3 Grubb A. Commentary on Re B. Medical Law Review 2002; 10:203.

Chapter 8

The impact of the Human Rights Act 1998 on health care in the UK

Richard Burchill

'Health is a fundamental human right indispensable for the exercise of other human rights. Every human being is entitled to the enjoyment of the highest attainable standard of health conducive to living a life in dignity.'[1]

INTRODUCTION

To say that individuals have a 'right to health' is not necessarily a controversial claim. However, trying to ensure that all individuals enjoy the highest attainable standard of health raises numerous practical difficulties as resources are finite and the needs of all individuals will not always be met. The dilemmas faced in trying to meet the demands inherent in ensuring the right to health, centre on competing claims of the needs of society on the one hand and the particular needs of individuals on the other. The result is that debates about the right to health focus primarily on the economic issues of how much and for whom healthcare resources will be allocated. Too often in this debate the normative or human rights issues relating to healthcare provision are ignored. A primary reason why human rights issues are marginalised is that it is consistently believed that questions involving healthcare policy and human rights are not amenable to any sort of judicial resolution and are better left for the elected politicians to decide. But given the controversial or difficult decisions inherent in questions over health care and human rights, the elected legislature should not be the exclusive forum for this debate.[2]

The passage of the Human Rights Act 1998 (HRA) provides the opportunity for greater emphasis to be placed on the human rights side of the discussion about healthcare provision. The HRA allows for most of the rights contained in the European Convention on Human Rights (ECHR) to be directly actionable before UK courts. It also places an obligation upon public authorities to act in a manner consistent with the ECHR. More importantly, the HRA requires the judiciary to deal directly with human rights questions before it, even if it involves questions about policy and economic resources. The UK judiciary has consistently and explicitly avoided dealing with human rights issues when faced with questions that the judiciary has considered involve matters of healthcare policy. The judiciary's constant deference to Parliament is overly simplistic and inadequate in the context of health care.[3] By addressing the human rights implications in healthcare policy the judiciary would be making a significant contribution by allowing for greater discussion and debate about the adequacies of government policy.

This contribution will examine how the HRA provides the opportunity, if not a mandate, for the judiciary to take on a new role when questions about human rights and health care are before the courts. It will not be suggested that the judiciary should be allowed to decide specific matters of healthcare policy: that will remain the responsibility of the elected policy makers and administrators.

HEALTHCARE RIGHTS PRIOR TO THE HRA

Before the passage of the HRA the UK did not possess a 'positive' system for human rights protection. The protection of rights depended upon developments in the common law and through construing the existence of a right in statutory provisions. Rights, or more appropriately, liberties, were conceived in negative terms whereby individuals were free to act unless there existed a specific limitation on individual liberty. The UK's constitutional system is based on the idea that Parliament is the supreme authority and the judiciary must defer to the express will of Parliament, with limited weight given to the impact of a particular law upon individual rights. Even though the UK is party to a wide range of European and international human rights instruments, which declare the existence of positive rights for the individual and demand that governments respect and ensure these rights, the ability of individuals to claim the existence of positive rights in the domestic system has been severely limited.

This is not to say that the UK offered no possibility for the protection of human rights. Rights protection did exist prior to the HRA and judges did, in a rather haphazard way, try to further the protection of human rights in cases before them.[4] However, given the strongly held views that the judiciary must defer to the expressed will of Parliament, much of the support for rights prior to the HRA has been accurately described as 'deviation and dissent' from the overall development of the UK constitution where rights protection has been described as being in a state of crisis.[5] This was especially the case with socio-economic rights, an attitude that continues today. Socio-economic rights are commonly considered to be goals or targets to be achieved incrementally over time as they involve major financial and policy considerations. Since, it is believed, these rights are dependent upon policy they are also not amenable to positive enforcement by the courts and questions over rights when resources or policy are in question are commonly considered to be non-justiciable matters.[6]

The UK judiciary, in common with judges in many legal systems, has consistently attempted to avoid judgments that involve engaging with policy making. The basis for the judiciary's stance is embedded in a particular belief in the separation of powers. This belief holds that Parliament, as the elected representatives of society, is best placed to make and implement socio-economic policy. The judiciary, as an unelected body, should not become involved in matters of policy. Accordingly, the only role for the courts is to ensure that administrative power is exercised in a fair and reasonable manner. When faced with a situation where the implementation of what are considered policy decisions have given rise to alleged human rights violations, the judiciary has confined itself to examining only how the decision was made and has veered away from engaging with the substance or result of the decision. As Lord Denning explained 'The Secretary of State says that he is doing the best he can with the financial resources available to him: and I don't think he can be faulted in the matter' (R v. *Secretary of State for Social Services, West Midlands RHA and Birmingham AHA*, ex p. *Hincks* [1980] 1 BMLR 93). Lord Denning made it clear that the court could not question the decisions made by the Secretary of State in relation to how resources were allocated, regardless of the impact those decisions may have had.

The dilemmas faced by the judiciary prior to the HRA are illustrated in the well-known case of R v. *Cambridge Health Authority*, ex p. *B* [1995] 1 FLR 1055. Before the High Court, consideration was given to the impact upon human rights of a policy decision, but the Court of Appeal refused to entertain the substance of the human rights issues and took a deferential position on what it considered to be policy decisions. B had been diagnosed with leukaemia and the Cambridge Health Authority would not provide the funding for further treatment that it believed was clinically unproven. Before the High Court Laws J made his view clear, declaring 'Of all human rights, most people would accord the most precious place to the right to life itself'. Laws J admitted that the court could not make clinical decisions, but since the fundamental right to life was engaged it could not just restrict itself to determining if the decision not to provide treatment was a reasonable one or not. The basis for his position was that 'certain rights, broadly those occupying a central place in the [ECHR] and obviously including the right to life, are not to be perceived as moral or political aspirations nor as enjoying a legal status only upon the international plane …. . They are to be vindicated as sharing with other principles the substance of the English common law.'

Laws J maintained that it is up to the public authority to make the necessary decision, and the courts are obliged to recognise the power conferred by

Parliament. However, he also asserted that when a public authority is before the courts 'the decision-maker has to recognise that he can only infringe such a fundamental right by virtue of an objection of substance put forward in the public interest'. Laws J did not accept that if the health authority simply 'toll[ed] the bell of tight resources' the court had to accept it unquestioningly.

The case immediately went to the Court of Appeal, which overturned the decision of Laws J, primarily on the basis that he had gone too far in asserting the role of the judiciary in cases of this nature. In giving the opinion of the Court of Appeal, Bingham MR started with the position that 'Our society is one in which a very high value is put on human life. No decision affecting human life is one that can be regarded with other than the greatest seriousness.' It is important to note that this starting proposition was not the same as Laws J: Bingham MR made no reference to the individual's right to life, saying only that life is of high value.[7] As Bingham MR's position did not place the human rights of the individual as a primary consideration he disagreed with the overall approach of Laws J. Bingham MR felt it would be 'totally unrealistic' for the courts to require that a health authority explain its decision. Bingham MR's position was clearly based on the belief that matters of funding involve policy decisions and that the judiciary does not have a role to play in such matters even if human rights are involved. Since it was believed that such matters involved questions which the elected Parliament was more competent to deal with the plea of tight resources was a good enough explanation for the courts.[3]

Bingham MR's position is in line with the general views of the judiciary. It has been said that the courts cannot 'enhance the standards of the National Health Service' and that the courts have 'no role of general investigator of social policy and of allocation of resources' (*R* v. *Central Birmingham HA, ex p. Collier* 6 January 1988, unreported). It has been felt that these were matters solely for Parliament to consider (*Airedale NHS Trust* v. *Bland* [1993] 2 WLR 316; *Wilsher* v. *Essex AHA* [1987] 2 WLR 425) and crucially, that any questions about the impact of policy decisions were 'to be raised, answered and dealt with outside the courts' (*R* v. *Central Birmingham HA* ex p. *Walker* [1987] 3 BMLR 32). The courts have generally recognised the gravity of applications before them when fundamental human rights are involved, but at the same time they have remained confined to examining the process of decision making and not the substantive impact of the decision. It is submitted that the approach of Laws J, discussed above, should be seen as appropriate for proper consideration was given to the importance of human rights but at the same time the court was not attempting to make decisions about policy. Laws J was trying to expand the debate about how policy decisions impact upon human rights in order to give appropriate consideration to the importance of human rights.

THE IMPACT OF THE HUMAN RIGHTS ACT

Many commentators have acknowledged that the HRA will have a significant impact in the field of health care.[8–12] In a speech given when the HRA first entered into force, the then Lord Chancellor, Lord Irvine, raised the question as to the extent to which the HRA would be relevant to the medical field. His response was 'more than you might guess'.[13] The Lord Chancellor has also explained that the system for the protection of human rights prior to the HRA was not sufficient as it 'offer[ed] little protection against a creeping erosion of freedom by a legislature willing to countenance infringement of liberty or simply blind to the effect of an otherwise well intentioned piece of law'.[14] He has further expressed the hope that the HRA would work to promote a culture where positive rights are given proper concern by legislators, administrators and judges.[14] Now with a positive system of human rights protection in place the judiciary, when faced with human rights questions, is obliged to concentrate more on issues of substance rather than form, giving proper consideration to the normative questions involved.

The HRA does not necessarily mark a major revolution in the constitutional system, as it keeps in place the supreme position of Parliament. At the same time the HRA provides for new opportunities to ensure the effective protection of human rights. Section 3 places an interpretative obligation upon the courts whereby '[s]o far as it is possible to do so, primary legislation and subordinate legislation must be read and given effect in a way which is compatible with Convention rights'. Section 2 provides that 'A court or tribunal determining a question which has arisen in connection with the Convention right must take into account any' judgment, decision, declaration or opinion given under the ECHR. By 'taking into account' the jurisprudence from Strasbourg, the courts will not be bound by the decisions of the European Court of Human Rights (ECtHR). The purpose behind this wording is to ensure that developments in the protection of human rights through the common law and through domestic statutes are preserved. At the same time it is an opportunity for the courts to take a more outward view and make use of the wide range of international human rights instruments beyond the ECHR. Section 6 requires all public authorities to act in a manner which is compatible with the majority of rights set out in the ECHR, as included in Schedule 1 of the HRA.

None of the rights in Schedule 1 directly addresses a right to health or a right to health care. However, a range of ECHR rights included in Schedule 1 have been identified as having an impact upon health care, such as Article 2 – right to life; Article 3 – prohibition of cruel, inhuman or degrading treatment; Article 5 – right to liberty and security; Article 6 – right to a fair trial; Article 8 – right to respect for family and private life; Article 10 – right to freedom of expression which has included a right to information; and Article 14 – the prohibition of discrimination in relation to any right in the ECHR.

The rights contained in the ECHR possess different levels of obligations depending upon the nature of the right in question. Articles 2 and 3 are considered absolute rights where violations can only be justified in the most limited of circumstances, if at all. Restriction on the rights contained in Articles 5 and 6 are legitimate in specific circumstances as set out in those provisions. Articles 8 and 10 often require the balancing of competing interests to determine if a specific limitation is acceptable. It has been widely suggested that the judiciary will now be actively engaging in interpretation based upon proportionality where it must be determined whether or not the objective which is being sought justifies limiting human rights, whether the means chosen are appropriate, and whether these means are the least invasive upon rights (*de Freitas* v. *Permanent Secretary of Ministry of Agriculture, Fisheries, Lands and Housing* [1998] 3 WLR 675).

It is well recognised that when it comes to interpretation of human rights instruments the judiciary will not use the normal rules of statutory interpretation. It has been explained that the ECHR 'should be seen as an expression of fundamental principles rather than as a set of mere rules' (*R* v. *DPP*, ex p. *Kebilene* [1999] 3 WLR 972). Other jurisdictions, which have constitutional instruments for the protection of human rights, provide examples as to how the UK judiciary needs to approach human rights interpretation. The interpretation of the Canadian Charter of Fundamental Rights and Freedoms has been described as 'a generous rather than legalistic one, aimed at fulfilling the purpose of the guarantees and securing for individuals the full benefit of the Charter's protection' (*R* v. *Big M Drug Mart* [1985] 1 SCR 295). It has been stated that the New Zealand Bill of Rights Act should be given 'such fair, large and liberal construction and interpretation as will best ensure the attainment of its object according to its true intent, meaning and spirit' (*Ministry of Transport* v. *Noort* [1992] 3 NZLR 260). The Privy Council has also expressed the importance of interpreting constitutional rights provisions in a different way, ensuring that full recognition and respect is given to human rights protection (*Minister of Foreign Affairs* v. *Fisher* [1979] 2 WLR 889). It is essential that instruments protecting human rights are given their full import even if judicial decisions are not necessarily popular with either government or society.[15]

The main problem facing the judiciary is treading a fine line between interpretation and legislation (*Poplar Housing and Regeneration Community Association Ltd* v. *Donoghue* [2001] 3 WLR 183). UK judges are well aware of the separation of powers doctrine and are careful about overstepping the mark and engaging in any form of legislating.[16] But at the same time, the judiciary can no longer remain aloof from human rights issues. With the HRA the judiciary can no longer simply defer to Parliament on the basis of a policy matter if issues of human rights are engaged, since the HRA 'must be given its full import and … long or well entrenched ideas may have to be put aside, sacred cows culled' (*R* v. *Lambert* [2001] 3 WLR 206). It is clear that the sacred cow of judicial deference in matters of socio-economic policy involving questions of human rights has to be culled. The ECtHR has said that it is necessary to interpret the ECHR so that rights are not just 'theoretical or illusory' but rather to ensure that they are 'practical and effective' (*Airey* v. *Ireland* [1979] 2 EHRR 305).

JUSTICIABLE NATURE OF SOCIO-ECONOMIC RIGHTS

One of the major effects of the HRA upon healthcare rights is that matters which the judiciary used to consider to be beyond their competence, or non-justiciable, the courts must now address. Studies have shown that many domestic courts have recognised the justiciable nature of healthcare rights in countries like Italy, Poland, Colombia, Brazil, Thailand, India and South Africa.[17,18] The South African example is especially intriguing as this is a country which possesses constitutionally enshrined socio-economic rights including the right to health care but suffers severe poverty.[19] Nonetheless, the judiciary has treated these rights as justiciable matters and not solely as a concern of the elected legislature.[20]

Viewing matters of health care and human rights as justiciable is not as radical as it may appear: it merely brings the UK in line with its international human rights obligations. The UK has been a party to the International Covenant on Economic Social and Cultural Rights (ICESCR) since 1976. The ICESCR contains a range of socio-economic rights including Article 12 which provides for 'the right of everyone to the highest attainable standard of physical and mental health'. Under the ICESCR the rights contained therein are to be met in a programmatic fashion which leads many, especially governments, to conclude that these rights are non-justiciable.[6] The monitoring body for the ICESCR, the Economic and Social Council (ECOSOC) strongly disagrees with the position that the rights in the ICESCR are non-justiciable. ECOSOC recognises the programmatic nature of the rights in ICESCR but it also emphasises that concrete measures are to be taken and among these measures judicial remedies are appropriate.[21] In a specific statement to the UK, ECOSOC has explained that it 'finds disturbing the position of the State party that provisions of the Covenant, with certain minor exceptions, constitute principles and programmatic objectives rather than legal obligations …'.[22] ECOSOC has suggested that the UK 'take appropriate steps to introduce into legislation the International Covenant …, so that the rights covered by the Covenant may be fully implemented' and due regard be given to the UK's obligations under the ICESCR.[22]

Incorporating the UK's international human rights obligations into the domestic system would give the judiciary a stronger role as the protector of rights and helps to ensure full consideration is given to human rights issues. It would also assist in helping to ensure that the right to health is realised since Article 12 of the ICESCR requires a state to take 'deliberate, concrete and targeted steps' for ensuring that this right is met.[1] Such an obligation obviously means that the government needs to take positive actions, which in turn will have implications for economic policy. This is a major reason why the UK judiciary has been reluctant to become involved in these matters (*Re J* [1992] 3 WLR 507). Commentators have noted that domestic courts tend only to deal with the minimum core content of healthcare rights, leaving anything above this core to the discretion of the government.[17] In the UK context, even if courts confine themselves to the idea of a minimum core they will have a significant impact as to what constitutes the extent to which positive action is necessary to ensure that the rights are protected.[6]

The idea that governments are under an obligation to engage in positive action for the protection of rights is also recognised in ECHR jurisprudence. In *Association X* v. *UK* [1978] 14 DR 31 it was stated that Article 2 ECHR requires the state not to take life and also 'to take the appropriate steps to safeguard life'. In *Tanko* v. *Finland* (Application No. 23634/94 (19 May 1994)) it was said that 'a lack of proper care in a case where someone is suffering from a serious illness could in certain circumstances amount to treatment contrary to Article 3'. In the case of *LCB* v. *UK* [1998] 27 EHRR 212 the ECtHR reiterated that the right to life in Article 2 imposes obligations on the state to prevent human life being avoidably put at risk, as the government is under an obligation 'to take appropriate steps to safeguard the lives of those within its jurisdiction ...'. In *D* v. *UK* [1997] 24 EHRR 423 the ECtHR felt that if the government could prevent the suffering attributable to the progression of a fatal disease then the failure to take such positive action could be considered a violation of Article 3. It should be noted that the positive obligation on states is not absolute. The ECtHR in *Osman* v. *UK* [2000] 29 EHRR 245 repeated that states have a positive obligation to ensure that rights are realised, but this obligation was limited to ensuring only that which is possible and must not place a disproportionate burden on the government. When assessing the positive obligations upon a state there is the need to take into account all relevant considerations as the requirements will vary considerably depending upon the given situation (*Rees* v. *UK* [1986] 9 EHRR 56).

It is clear that the UK government is under an obligation through international human rights law to ensure that individuals are able to realise their rights to health. This places a clear duty on the government to take the necessary measures to ensure access to health facilities, goods and services so that individuals may be able to enjoy the highest attainable standard of health.[1] Where limitations are placed on healthcare rights these can only be justified when they are compatible with the larger concept of effective human rights protection; when they are in the interest of legitimate aims being pursued; when they are strictly necessary for the promotion of general welfare in a democratic society; or when they are proportional and only to the extent necessary.[1] ECOSOC considers that an essential element for ensuring the above standards are met is a favourable environment for the protection of healthcare rights, based on principles of accountability, transparency, and an independent judiciary.[1] The role of the judiciary in ensuring that a government effectively meets its obligations with regard to health care is very important.[18] In *LCB* v. *UK* the ECtHR explained that the task of the judiciary is to 'determine whether, given the circumstances of the case, the State did all that could have been required of it to prevent the applicant's life from being avoidably put at risk'. The judiciary cannot simply defer or claim that the matter is non-justiciable.

Admittedly, for a range of reasons, judges are perhaps not best placed to make clinical decisions or to decide how public money is spent, but at the same time they do and can play a constructive role in questions about health care when human rights are involved.[19] In *Marcic* v. *Thames Water Utilities Ltd.* [2002] 2 WLR 932, a case involving not health care but socio-economic concerns, it was argued that the court was not the appropriate body for making technical decisions or for deciding how competing interests should be balanced. The court held, referring to the decision in *ex parte B*, that since an individual's human rights were in question, it was perfectly appropriate for the court to enter into the substance of the case. Such statements are rare. The judiciary generally relies on the statement given in *ex parte Kebilene* where the appropriate role of the courts was explained:

> 'difficult choices may have to be made by the executive or the legislature between the rights of the individual and the needs of society. In some circumstances it will be appropriate for the courts to recognise that there is an area of judgment within which the judiciary will defer, on democratic grounds, to the considered opinion of the elected body or person whose act or decision is said to be incompatible with the Convention ... where the area in which these choices may arise is conveniently and appropriately described as the "discretionary area of judgment". It will be easier for such an area of judgment to be recognised where the Convention itself requires a balance to be struck, much less so where the right is stated in terms which are unqualified. It will be easier for it to be recognised where the issues involve questions of social or economic policy, much less so where the rights are of high constitutional importance or are of a kind where the courts are especially well placed to assess the need for protection.'

The court in *Kebilene* stated that areas of socio-economic policy fall clearly within the 'discretionary area of judgment' and, on such matters, the judiciary will defer to Parliament. In the recent case involving Dianne Pretty the court explained that difficult decisions need to be made in areas where there is no broad agreement and the courts will leave it up to the democratically elected decision makers and not through 'judicial creativity' (*R (on the application of Pretty)* v. *DPP (HL)* [2001] 3 WLR 1598).

This is indicative of the problem facing human rights protection in the UK, where the judiciary remains strongly deferential to Parliament on the premise that the courts should not be involved in political decisions. The judiciary's active maintenance of its deferential position to Parliament so as to avoid politics, is itself a political statement about the role of the courts in the UK.[19] Taking human rights questions to the courts should not be seen as challenging administrators or overstepping perceived constitutional boundaries established by the separation of powers. Instead it needs to be seen as one possible means of strengthening the decision making process.[23] To suggest that greater attention be given to human rights as a matter of substantial concern for the courts is not to force judges into an unacceptable realm of judicial creativity. Rather it is to move them into their rightful position as guardians of human rights, ensuring that the UK meets the various obligations it has agreed to. As Lord Woolf[15] has explained, there will be times when 'Parliament or the government will not strike the correct balance between the rights of society as a whole and the rights of the individual'. It is in these situations that the judges will have to say where the correct balance lies. In cases involving health care since the adoption of the HRA, the judiciary has shown a tendency to be overly concerned with the meaning of words or phrases and in trying to demonstrate that the common law and past decisions are compatible with the HRA. The result has been that the broad principles inherent in human rights protection have not been given their full importance.[24,25] Ominously, in *North West*

Lancashire HA v. *A, D and G* [2000] 1 WLR 977, the court stated that human rights should not be argued in a case involving treatment in gender reassignment, even though the essential issue at stake was one of human dignity, which is the essential purpose behind human rights.

CONCLUSION

The importance of the judiciary actively engaging in human rights questions related to health policy is undeniable. As the statement of ECOSOC quoted at the beginning of this chapter makes clear – the right to health is fundamental and is indispensable for the exercise of other human rights and all individuals are entitled to high standards of health essential to living a life of dignity. So far, the HRA has not substantially changed the nature or degree of human rights protection in health care. Judges have been reluctant to dip 'their toes into the largely uncharted waters of the Human Rights Act'.[9] There is also evidence of an unfortunate lack of knowledge about the HRA in some areas of the public services.[26] The discussion above demonstrates that the UK's international obligations and the underlying nature and purpose of the HRA, demand that the judiciary abandons its traditional reluctance to become involved in socio-economic matters, and its traditional deference to Parliament in these matters. At the very least it is necessary to recognise that health care and human rights are significantly related:

> 'What human rights does for public health is to provide an internally agreed upon framework for setting out the responsibilities of government under human rights law as these relate to people's health and welfare.'[27]

The HRA does this by providing a tool for service users which, properly used, will help to ensure their human rights are fully taken into account in making decisions about access to treatment and services.[9] Gruskin and Tarantola[18] observe '[h]uman rights are progressively being understood to offer an approach for considering the broader societal dimensions and contexts of the well-being of individuals and populations, therefore to be of utility to all of those concerned with health'.

Lord Irvine[13] has noted that the HRA 'will gradually reshape the climate' in which courts deal with human rights. Part of this is due to society becoming more amenable to litigation, but also it can be attributed to individuals becoming more aware of their human rights and demanding that the government respect these rights. Others have noted that it is likely that claims of violations involving health rights will increase both at the national and international level.[18] If the judiciary continues to defer to Parliament in matters of health care and refuses to become actively involved when human rights are at stake, it appears that the hopes that the HRA will create a culture of rights in the UK will not be realised. The burden is not only on the judiciary; it is also up to lawyers and other professionals involved in health care to be aware of and fully recognise the importance of human rights. ECOSOC has criticised the UK for not sufficiently informing the public and others about obligations under the ICESCR with the result that 'judges and other members of the legal profession have not given sufficient consideration to the importance of this Covenant within domestic law'.[28] Lord Woolf[15] has explained that 'The Human Rights Act has strengthened our democracy by giving each member of the public the right to seek the help of the courts to protect his or her human rights in a manner that was not previously available'. It is now up to the judiciary to recognise its role and act upon it.

References

1   ECOSOC (United Nations Economic and Social Council). General Comment No. 14. UN Doc. E/C.12/2000/4; 2000: paras 1, 28, 30, 53, 55.
2   Kennedy I, Grubb A. Medical law, 3rd edn. London: Butterworths; 2000:45.
3   Whitty N. In a perfect world: feminism and healthcare resource allocation. In: Sheldon S, Thomson M, eds. Feminist perspectives on healthcare law. London: Cavendish; 1998:135–153.
4   Hunt M. Using Human Rights Law in English Courts. Oxford: Hart; 1997:Chs 4–7.
5   Ewing KD, Gearty CA. Freedom under Thatcher: civil liberties in modern Britain. Oxford: Oxford University Press; 1990:255.
6   Craven M. The justiciability of economic, social and cultural rights. In: Burchill R, Harris D, Owers A, eds. Economic, social and cultural rights: their implementation in United Kingdom law. Nottingham: University of Nottingham Human Rights Law Centre; 1999:1–13.
7   O'Sullivan D. The allocation of scarce resources and the right to life under the European convention on human rights. Public Law 1998; Autumn:389–395.
8   Brahams D. Impact of European Human Rights Law. Lancet 2000; 21 October:1433–1434.
9   Haggett E. The Human Rights Act 1998 and access to NHS treatments and services: a practical guide. London: The Constitution Unit; 2001:7.
10 Hewson B. Why the Human Rights Act matters to doctors. British Medical Journal 2000; 321:780–781.
11 Horton R. Health and the UK Human Rights Act 1998. Lancet 2000; 356: 1186–1188.
12 English V, Romano-Critchley G, Sommervill A, et al. Ethics briefing. Journal of Medical Ethics 2000; 26:410.
13 Lord Irvine. The patient, the doctor, their lawyers and the judge: rights and duties. Medical Law Review 1999; 7(3):255–268.
14 Lord Irvine. The development of human rights in Britain under an incorporated convention on human rights. Public Law 1998; Summer:221–236.
15 Lord Woolf. Human rights: have the public benefited? British Academy thanks-offering to Britain fund lecture 15 October 2002:3, 10, 11. Online. Available: www.britac.ac.uk/pubs/src/tob02/ 8 January 2003.
16 Lord Hoffmann. Human rights and the House of Lords. Modern Law Review 1999; 62(2):159–166.
17 Hendriks A. The right to health in national and international jurisprudence. European Journal of Health Law 1998; 5(4):389–408.

18 Gruskin S, Tarantola D. Health and human rights. Francois-Xavier Bagnoud Centre for Health and Human Rights Working Paper No. 10. 2000:14, 27. Online. Available: www.hsph.Harvard.edu/fxbcenter/working-papers.htm 8 January 2003.

19 van Buren G. Including the excluded: the case for an economic, social and cultural human rights act. Public Law 2002; Autumn:456–472.

20 Ngwena C. The recognition of access to health care as a human right in South Africa: is it enough? Health and Human Rights 2002; 5(1):27–44.

21 ECOSOC (United Nations Economic and Social Council). General Comment No. 3 UN Doc.E/1991/23, 1990; para 5.

22 ECOSOC (United Nations Economic and Social Council). Concluding observations of the Committee on economic, social and cultural rights: United Kingdom and Northern Ireland. UN Doc.E/C.12/1Add.19, 1997; paras 2.1, 10.

23 Syrett K. Nice work? Rationing, review and the 'legitimacy problem' in the new NHS. Medical Law Review 2002; 10(1):1–27.

24 Maclean AR. A crossing of the rubicon on the human rights ferry. Modern Law Review 2001; 64(5):775–794.

25 Palmer E. Resource allocation, welfare rights – mapping the boundaries of judicial control in public administrative law. Oxford Journal of Legal Studies 2000; 20(1):63–88.

26 Watson J. Something for everyone: the impact of the Human Rights Act and the need for a human rights commission. London: British Institute of Human Rights; 2002.

27 Tarantola D. Building on the synergy between health and human rights: a global perspective. Francois-Xavier Bagnoud Centre for Health and Human Rights Working Paper No. 8. 2000:1. Online. Available: www.hsph.Harvard.edu/fxbcenter/working-papers.htm 6 January 2003.

28 ECOSOC (United Nations Economic and Social Council). Concluding observations of the Committee on economic, social and cultural rights: United Kingdom and Northern Ireland. UN Doc. E/C.12/1994/19, 1994; para 8.

Further Reading

Den Exter A, Hermans H. The right to health care: a changing concept? In: Den Exter A, Hermans H, eds. The right to health care in several European countries. The Hague: Kluwer; 1999:1–10.

McHale J. Enforcing healthcare rights in the English courts. In: Burchill R, Harris D, Owers A, eds. Economic, social and cultural rights: their implementation in United Kingdom law. Nottingham: University of Nottingham Human Rights Law Centre; 1999:66–87.

Chapter **9**

How effective is the Human Rights Act 1998 in protecting genetic information?

Carolyn Johnston

UK BIOBANK

The Department of Health, working in partnership with the Wellcome Trust and the Medical Research Council has developed the UK Population Biomedical Collection, known as UK Biobank ('Biobank'). This is a national study that will consider the contribution of gene and environment interaction in the development of disease. The government considers Biobank to be the country's flagship project on molecular epidemiology for the new century. 'Biobank UK will provide a national resource for scientists wishing to study the interaction between genetic, environmental and lifestyle risk factors in the development of the common diseases of adult life, especially cardiovascular disease, metabolic disorders and cancer.'[i]

From the study of genetic data, medical histories and lifestyle/environment data it will be possible to establish whether particular medical conditions are associated with genetic features and in the future to produce drug therapies which are more effective by tailoring them to the needs of particular individuals. This is one of the objectives of the Biobank study.[1]

---

[i]Speech by Alan Milburn MP, then Secretary of State for Health at the international conference, Genetics and Health – A Decade of Opportunity, 16/1/2002.

It is proposed that 500 000 men and women volunteers between 45 and 69 years of age take part in the study.

Genetic and personal data on health and lifestyle will be taken by GPs from patients who have conditions which are of interest to the study, for example diabetes. There will be long-term follow up via NHS medical records to accumulate data on health outcomes. Research will be undertaken by 'spoke' groups of geneticists. A large amount of personal and sensitive information will be held in computerised databases (the 'hub') so that comparisons of samples can be made.

Genetic databases are not new. There are a number of existing collections of genetic information used for research[ii] and forensic purposes (National DNA Database). Additionally, NHS Regional Genetic Testing Centres carry out genetic testing on individuals who, by virtue of a family history, are considered to be at risk of a genetic disease.

In 1998 the parliament in Iceland passed legislation approving a DNA database project to study the genetic information of the 275 000 'pure-bred' residents of Iceland. A private company, deCODE Genetics, set up a database to use the genetic information of the majority of the population. To make the study workable there must be sufficient participants and this is achieved by presuming consent to use medical records unless individuals opt out. Approximately 11 500 residents have opted out so far. An opposition organisation called *Mannvernd* believes that the legislation infringes human rights and personal privacy.

The House of Lords Select Committee on Science and Technology ('Select Committee') considered the issues surrounding human genetic databases.[2] It highlighted the importance of British scientists and researchers making a contribution in this field, while recognising the need to effectively manage such personal and sensitive data. Obviously it is in the public interest that medical research continues, but in the aftermath of Alder Hey it is essential that the public supports, and has confidence in, research projects so that the undoubted benefits can be realised. Unless individuals can be assured that their genetic information is 'safe' and that there is adequate protection against misuse and disclosure it would be difficult to recruit them to the Biobank study. The linkage of genetic and health information and the potential for using the database for a wide variety of analyses aimed at determining susceptibility to disease raises important issues about confidentiality, security of data and informed consent.[iii]

But is research involving genetic information different from other medical research and should it have a greater level of protection? It could be argued that there is nothing special about genetic information[3] which distinguishes it from other health-related information – eye colour is genetic information but

---

[ii] For example, the Avon Longitudinal Study of Parents and Children, and the North Cumbria Community Genetics Project.

[iii] Speech by Alan Milburn MP, then Secretary of State for Health at the international conference, Genetics and Health – A Decade of Opportunity, 16/1/2002.

not deserving of special treatment. However, in its response to the Human Genetics Commission's discussion document, *Whose Hands on Your Genes?*, Liberty[4] considers that genetic information is special because of its peculiar intimacy, commercial value and the incentive for misuse of such information.[iv] Also it is easily obtainable (from a hair follicle, mouth swab or blood sample), can be stored indefinitely and is a uniquely personal identifier (except for identical twins). For practical purposes DNA cannot be anonymised. Information of genetic diseases has implications for family members as regards their susceptibility to disease.[v] By definition, hereditary diseases affect more than one person.

Where biobanks are concerned, potentially conflicting interests must be weighed against one another; interests of the participant, relatives, medical research and commercial interests and how far one interest is balanced against another is made more difficult with the rapid developments in genetic understanding.

In its report, *Inside Information* (May 2002),[5] the Human Genetics Commission (HGC) considers the balance of interests in the use of personal genetic information. Particular issues of concern, raised by GeneWatch UK[vi] and other interested parties are whether, and in what circumstances, access to genetic information held on genetic databases can be gained without consent of the participant and the potential for genetic discrimination by employers and insurers. As the science of behavioural genetics proceeds, the use of genetic information as a predictor for anti-social and criminal behaviour[6] assumes greater significance.

Here, it will be considered whether, and in what circumstances, genetic information may be disclosed to others without consent of the Biobank participant. Additionally, if during the Biobank study a medical researcher finds that a participant is at risk of a serious genetic disease, is Biobank under an *obligation* to disclose this information to the participant and/or his close relatives at risk?

The Select Committee recommended that the primary means of regulating human genetic databases should (continue to) be the Data Protection Act 1998 (DPA). There are, however, other ways to protect genetic information and the following is a consideration of the effectiveness of the DPA, the duty of confidentiality and more particularly the Human Rights Act 1998 (HRA) in protecting against non-consensual disclosure of genetic information held on the Biobank database.

[iv] DNA samples appear to be treated as 'information' rather than 'property' and legal principles applied accordingly. In respect of intellectual property rights in gene sequences, the Select Committee stated that 'we do not regard ownership of biological samples as a particularly useful concept with respect to human genetic databases. We prefer the notion of partnership between participants and researchers, for medical advance and the benefit of others, including future generations' (8.27).

[v] It is interesting to consider whether genetic diseases are caught by the NHS (Venereal Diseases) Regulations 1974 – they are sexually transmitted after all.

[vi] Giving Your Genes to Biobank UK: Questions to Ask, (December 2001), Online. Available: http://www.genewatch.org/HumanGen/Biobanks/FAQs.htm.

DATA PROTECTION ACT 1998[vii]

The HGC recognises that the DPA 'provides a strong legal basis to underpin the storage and disclosure of medical records'.[5] But does the DPA offer sufficient protection for genetic information?

The Data Protection Act 1998 (formerly 1984) was designed to implement Council Directive 95/46 concerning protection of an individual's personal data. The Directive states that 'Member States shall protect the *fundamental rights* and freedoms of natural persons and in particular their right to *privacy* with respect to the processing of personal data' (italics added). Although the human rights and privacy dimensions are clear from this statement these concepts are not stated anywhere in the DPA.

The DPA regulates the 'processing' of personal data held on a manual or computerised system.

'Personal data' is defined (s.1(1)) as information which would allow identification of a living individual. The Select Committee defined human genetic databases as collections of genetic sequence information, or of human tissue from which such information might be derived, that are or could be linked to named individuals.

It is proposed that data held by Biobank will be de-identified/anonymised. However, there has to be a means of linking genetic data back to the participant because the object of the study is to correlate genetic, lifestyle and disease information. As the information held on the Biobank database will allow relating back to a named individual the data are 'personal data' and come within the provisions of the DPA.

Special protections are afforded to 'sensitive personal data' (s.2), which includes information as to the physical or mental health or condition of an individual. The DPA does not distinguish between genetic and other data but the Select Committee noted that genetic information is considered to be particularly sensitive.

For the purposes of controlling use and disclosure of personal data the DPA creates 'data subjects' and 'data controllers'. A 'data subject' is a person who is the subject of personal data. Patients are data subjects, so too would be participants in Biobank. A 'data controller' is a person who determines the purposes and manner in which personal data are processed. Data controllers must notify and be registered with the Information Commissioner. Biobank will be a data controller.

Data controllers may only process data in accordance with the 'Data Protection Principles'. 'Processing' is given a very wide definition (s.1) and covers obtaining, holding, recording and disclosing the information.[7] Clearly then the research undertaken in the Biobank study will be caught by the provisions of the DPA – 'the analysis of genetic material that reveals information about a particular individual comes within the scope of the Act'.[8]

[vii]The Data Protection Act 1998 is amended by the Freedom of Information Act 2000, which provides for disclosure of information held by public authorities.

Some of the more important Data Protection Principles provide that personal data must be processed 'lawfully and fairly' (First Principle) and that technical measures are adequate to prevent unlawful processing, loss and damage of data (Seventh Principle). The latter is of particular importance given that the Biobank study will necessitate large computer databases.

Sensitive personal data can be processed only if a condition in Schedule 2 and a condition in Schedule 3 are satisfied.

Schedule 3, Condition 1, provides that the data subject has given 'explicit' consent to the processing. Medical researchers have underlined the importance that data from one research project be available to other researchers. The Select Committee report considered that provisions of the DPA could unduly hamper medical research if exchange of such data requires explicit consent. Now however, section 60 of the Health and Social Care Act 2001 provides that the Secretary of State may authorise the use of patient information for research purposes without seeking patient consent where seeking consent is impracticable (presumably this would apply to Biobank given the huge numbers of participants involved). The Health Service (Control of Patient Information) Regulations 2002 (in force on 1 June 2002) provide that: 'anything done ... that is necessary for the purpose of processing patient information in accordance with these Regulations shall be lawfully done despite any obligation of confidence owed by that person'. The regulations have been criticised as being 'extremely broad and provide even more opportunities for improper and unregulated use of patients' confidential data ...'.[9]

Use/disclosure of genetic information without consent

To what extent does the DPA allow disclosure of genetic information held in the Biobank database without consent of the participant?

Disclosure to family

If, in the course of the Biobank study, a researcher finds that a participant carries a disease gene, can that information be disclosed to family members if the individual does not consent to disclosure?

Schedule 3, Condition 3, provides that information may be processed (disclosed) to protect the 'vital interests' of another person where the individual has *unreasonably* withheld his consent to disclosure. 'Vital interests' are considered to be those essential to life – life-threatening circumstances. This would apply, for example, where an individual has a communicable disease and another person is in danger of infection. How relevant is this to the disclosure of genetic information?

Faulty genes may result in genetic disorders. Monogenic disorders (a fault in a single gene) are recessive or dominant. A recessive disorder (cystic fibrosis) occurs when an individual has a defective gene from each parent. If the individual has only one defective gene then he is an asymptomatic carrier of the disease. Dominant disorders require only one inherited gene to be defective.

How extreme the disease manifests itself depends on 'penetrance' – that is the individual susceptibility to it. Huntington's disease is a dominant monogenic disorder and the disease is considered almost inevitable, but typically of these types of disorders, is of late onset and indeed the age of onset may vary over several decades. Such diseases often have no cure but information that an individual carries the gene is statistically predictive of significant health effects and will allow informed reproductive and lifestyle choices.

However the majority of genetic diseases are not monogenic but multifactorial – that is the disease is a product of defective genes and individual susceptibility to external/lifestyle factors such as diet, smoking, exercise and stress. Breast cancer is a multifactorial disorder – genetic inheritance increases the risk but environmental factors play a part. Defects in the BRCA1 and BRCA2 genes result in 5–10% of breast and ovarian cancers but only 36–85% of women carrying the gene will develop breast cancer.[viii] The Biobank study will involve research into this type of genetic disease. Currently, it is difficult to predict the likelihood of developing the disease if the defective gene is present, but future medical development may provide a greater correlation between existence of the gene and manifestation of the disorder. Genetic testing can be used to confirm a diagnosis, predict later development of a disease and identify a carrier.

It is difficult to see how disclosure of genetic information without consent could be justified to protect 'vital interests'. Even if genetic information shows that an individual has a gene mutation for Huntington's disease, as the disease is late onset and currently not treatable it is not life-threatening in the sense that another's life is *immediately* at risk. Disclosure to a family member that he may carry the gene would not protect his vital interests because with current medical knowledge the disease is untreatable.

As there is a large environmental element in the development of many genetic diseases there would be insufficient correlation between the disclosure of genetic information and the protection of another person's interests.

Prevention or detection of crime

Personal data may be processed (disclosed, used) without consent if it is necessary for the administration of justice, prevention or detection of any unlawful act (Data Protection (Processing of Sensitive Personal data) Order 2000).

In the case of *Campbell* v. *MGN Ltd* [2002] EWHC 499 the High Court considered that information about the therapy the model was receiving at Narcotics Anonymous was 'sensitive personal information' and was protected from disclosure unless there was a justification under the Act. A justification would be the prevention of crime. The Court referred to the fact that disclosure in this case was not in connection with drugs offences – if it was then perhaps there would be justification to disclose. On appeal the Court of

---

[viii] GeneWatch UK, Genetic testing in insurance and employment: a new form of discrimination, Briefing Number 15, June 2001, Online. Available: http://www.genewatch.org.

Appeal ([2002] EWCA 1373) found that the defendant could invoke section 32, which allowed processing of personal data for journalistic publishing in the public interest. However, this exemption could not be used to justify the publication of genetic information of participants in Biobank. The HGC has recommended the consideration of a criminal offence of non-consensual or deceitful obtaining of personal genetic information for non-medical purposes.[10]

Section 10 of the DPA provides that a data subject can prevent processing of his personal data that is likely to cause damage or distress. Information given to relatives of their risk of a genetic disease, without consent of the participant in Biobank, could be shown to cause distress to the participant. However section 10 does not apply where information is to be disclosed to protect the vital interests of an individual or for the administration of justice!

In its response to the HGC's discussion document, *Whose Hands on Your Genes?*, Liberty considered that 'existing legislation and codes of professional conduct have not been drafted with an eye to protecting genetic information'.[11] It suggested the introduction of statute and delegated legislation (to be under the control of an independent regulatory authority, along the lines of the Human Fertilisation and Embryology Authority) covering all those holding personal genetic information.

Indeed it is surprising that an Act drafted so recently should not have any reference, or particular relevance to genetic information. The office of the Information Commissioner has previously indicated that there is insufficient expertise to judge whether any particular processing of genetic information is acceptable.[ix] The Human Genetics Commission considered whether fair processing of genetic information could only be achieved by specific legislation.[x] In its report, the HGC recognised that 'there is considerable ambiguity in the precise application of current laws and that breach of Data Protection Principles is not a criminal offence'.[12]

CONFIDENTIALITY

The duty of confidentiality arises when information which is not publicly known is entrusted to a person in circumstances imposing an obligation not to disclose it, without the authority of the person who imparted it. Confidentiality arises because of the circumstances in which the information is imparted.

The duty of confidence has long been used to protect confidential medical information.

There is a public interest in maintaining confidentiality of medical information; health professionals need their patients to give them full and accurate information in order to treat them properly and patients may not do so without

---

[ix] Written Evidence to the House of Lords Select Committee on Science and Technology, Session 1999–2000 'Letter from the Office of the Data Protection Commissionery' 18 October 2000.
[x] At the HGC meeting of 20 November 2002, the Medical Research Council stated that it would seek counsel's opinion as to whether the DPA would enable a participant to have access to his genetic information held by Biobank.

assurances that these details will be kept confidential (*X* v. *Y and others* [1988] 2 All ER 648). If a patient did not think his details would be kept confidential he might not seek medical treatment (and indeed it would be difficult to recruit participants for Biobank).

If an individual undergoes genetic testing at a Regional Genetic Centre (because there is a risk that he carries a genetic mutation) there will be a doctor/patient relationship with the genetic therapist. The genetic information disclosed is certainly subject to the duty of confidence; it is given in circumstances where confidence should be respected and the nature of the information is recognised to be covered by the duty.

By comparison there is no doctor/patient relationship between the participant in Biobank and the medical researcher looking for a link between genes and lifestyle/environmental factors of many hundreds of samples. However, there is no requirement of a pre-existing confidential relationship in order to establish a duty of confidence.

In *Stephens* v. *Avery* [1988] 2 WLR 1280, the court said 'the relationship between the parties is not the determining factor. It is the acceptance of the information on the basis that it will be kept secret that affects the conscience of the recipient of the information' (per Sir Nicholas Browne-Wilkinson VC at 1268).

Therefore information held on the Biobank database will be subject to the duty of confidence despite the fact that there is no doctor/patient relationship between the participant and the researchers.

The data that Biobank will hold are to be de-identified (anonymised). Anonymised information is frequently used in the NHS for research purposes. Is such information subject to an obligation of confidence? In the case of *R* v. *Dept of Health* ex p. *Source Informatics* [1999] 52 BMLR 65, [2000] 1 All ER 786, the Court of Appeal held that prescription information which did not include the name of the patient (which was to be supplied by pharmacists to Source Informatics for analysis of the prescribing habits of GPs) was not subject to an obligation of confidence because individuals could not be identified.[xi] The difference with the data to be held by Biobank is that it will be possible to link the data with a named individual by way of a code held by an identified person (a trusted third party).[xii] As a result data held by Biobank will not fall within the Source Informatics exception.

When, if at all, can confidential information be disclosed?

An individual may of course *consent* to disclosure of confidential information. Sometimes it is implied from the circumstances that consent has been given. For example, information is passed to members of a medical treating team on

---

[xi] The 'conscience test' considered by Simon Brown LJ – 'would a reasonable pharmacist's conscience be troubled by the proposed use to be made of patient's prescriptions?' – may have been displaced by the decision of the Court of Appeal in the case of *LRT* v. *Mayor of London*, 24 August 2001 (unreported).

[xii] The effectiveness of encryption of genetic information held on the Biobank database was considered by the HGC (evidence R. Anderson) 19 November 2002.

a 'need to know basis'. All members of the team will be bound by the duty of confidentiality.[xiii]

It is recognised that there is a benefit for the genetic services in exchanging information. There would be no breach of the duty of confidence if an individual was informed of this and consented and indeed the Select Committee considered that consent could be implied for these purposes if the individual had been informed of potential uses for his genetic information.

Obviously a participant in Biobank may consent to his genetic information being used for other research programmes. The primary use by Biobank of the genetic information will be for the purpose of research into gene/disease correlation. Consideration has been given to secondary use of such data (presumably a variety of genetic research projects) and the extent to which a participant is required to give consent for this. The Select Committee recognised that secondary analysis of data is a 'vital part of the public health function' although the Medical Research Council has noted the potential for unforeseen experiments on retained samples.

The duty of confidentiality is not absolute and there may be circumstances where even though an individual refuses to consent to disclosure there are other interests that outweigh the refusal.

In *Campbell* v. *MGN Ltd* [2002] All ER (D) 448 (Mar) the High Court found there was a breach of the duty of confidence. Naomi Campbell's attendance at meetings of Narcotics Anonymous had the 'necessary quality of confidence about them' (photographs were taken surreptitiously when the model was obviously attending her private business) and disclosure of these details was not in the substantial public interest. However on appeal, the Court of Appeal[xiv] found that the information that she was receiving treatment from Narcotics Anonymous was not to be equated with disclosure of clinical details of medical treatment. Therefore the publication of such information was not sufficiently significant to amount to breach of confidence.

Concern has been raised at the possibility that the police could access data held on the Biobank database.[xv] In Scotland, a prisoner, Stephen Kelly,[xvi] volunteered to take part in an HIV study. All participants were assured that the findings would be kept confidential. However, later his sample was used as evidence in a criminal trial and he was convicted of knowingly infecting his girlfriend (who had taken part in a separate research project). The guarantee of confidentiality was overridden by the court in the public interest, i.e. that serious crime should be effectively investigated and prosecuted.

[xiii] Department of Health Protection and Use of Patient Information 1996 states that all NHS and non NHS staff working in healthcare settings are subject to the same common law duty of confidentiality.

[xiv] *Campbell* v. *MGN Ltd* [2002] EWCA Civ 1373. Naomi Campbell had conceded that only the publishing of information of her attendance at Narcotics Anonymous meetings and not that she had a drug problem, amounted to a breach of confidence.

[xv] GeneWatch UK. Evidence to the Science and Technology Committee, MRC November 2002.

[xvi] *Her Majesty's Advocate* v. *Stephen Robert Kelly* [2001] Scot HC7, 20 February 2001.

In order to give confidence to participants in Biobank that their donated material would be 'safe' and could not be interfered with by the police, the HGC thought it appropriate to ask the Home Secretary to make a statement to this effect in the House.[xvii] However, as discussed above, the DPA does allow information to be disclosed for the prevention/detection of a crime. The duty of confidentiality is never absolute and police investigating serious crimes can obtain court orders forcing health professionals to disclose information.

Disclosure in the health interests of family members

Genetic research has implications for the individual and his relatives as regards their susceptibility to disease. It is most usual for genetic information to be willingly shared between family members so that others may be tested and treated where appropriate. However, an individual may be reluctant to do so – the genetic condition may be severe, of late onset and with no effective treatment and there may be concerns of genetic discrimination by insurers and employers. Are there any circumstances when disclosure of an individual's genetic status to his family members for their benefit may be justified without the individual's consent?

The Genetics Interest Group considered the possibility that where a patient undergoes genetic testing at a Regional Genetic Centre there could be an agreement between the genetic services and the patient that he would voluntarily accept the obligation to assist other members of his family. It concluded however that this would be unnecessarily coercive.[13]

In considering whether to breach confidentiality, a balance is to be made between the potential harm to the individual in breaching confidentiality (harm to family relationships, especially if others were required to make difficult choices regarding reproduction) and whether this would be outweighed by the benefit to the relative of being informed (preventative measures/treatment could be undertaken).

GMC guidelines (Confidentiality: Protecting and Providing Information 2000) state that only in exceptional circumstances should information be disclosed against the wishes of a patient. 'Exceptional' cases include those where the health and safety of others is at serious risk, where there is an identifiable threat of harm presented by the patient. These guidelines have been recognised by the court (W v. Egdell [1990] 1 All ER 835), although it is not enough to have ethical guidelines if they are not effectively enforced.

Someone with a communicable disease may put others at risk by exposing them to infection. By comparison someone with disease genes does not himself put his relatives at risk – the risk of harm is a function of nature and family members will either have or not have the particular genetic makeup anyway. So a person with a genetic condition which could affect other members of his family is not posing a threat to them. The effect of the genetic inheritance may

---

[xvii] Meeting of HGC, 20 November 2002.

be ameliorated by warning them, but the threat itself is pre-existing and cannot be altered by the individual.

However, it is a relative's ignorance of being a carrier of the gene that poses a risk. Knowledge may allow plans to lessen the effect of future illness or to make reproductive choices. Early detection can prevent the cancer retinoblastoma. It is thought that a woman with the BRCA1 gene has about a 40% lifetime risk of getting breast cancer and this can increase to 80% in some high-risk families. Is this a sufficient risk to outweigh the importance of maintaining confidence? Would it make a difference if statistically there is a 90% chance that those with a genetic mutation would die before 35 years of age? In any event, it may be difficult to assess the precision with which test results predict the level of risk.

The BMA report, *Human Genetics: Choice and Responsibility*,[14] identifies certain factors which should be considered in deciding whether breach of confidence is justified: the severity of the disorder, the level of predictability of the information provided by testing, whether the condition is treatable and whether a relative is likely to be a carrier thereby affecting reproductive choices.

There should be a presumption against disclosure unless disclosure would avert a high probability of significant harm to an identifiable individual.

Liberty considers that allowing doctors or researchers to make the decision whether or not to disclose is 'too open to abuse'[xviii] and proposes that special permission should be obtained from a judge prior to disclosure.

Having balanced the issues for and against disclosure, the confidant (doctor, medical researcher) has a *discretion* to disclose. Could it ever be the case that there is an *obligation* at common law to disclose to family members at serious risk of genetic disease?

Obligation at common law to disclose serious risk of genetic disease?

In some states in the USA, there may be a duty on doctors to warn genetically 'at risk' relatives. In *Pate* v. *Threlkel* (661 So. 2d 278 [1995]), a patient received treatment for medullary thyroid carcinoma – a genetically transferable disease. The patient's daughter, although herself not a patient of that doctor, claimed that the failure to warn her of the risk meant that she did not seek early diagnosis and treatment and therefore developed advanced cancer. The special relationship with the patient imposed a duty to warn *family members* of an identifiable risk.

A geneticist working in a Regional Genetic Testing Centre could be considered to have a 'special relationship' with the individual whose genetic information he is testing as he is in a position to know of a risk not obvious to others. He is also in a position to prevent foreseeable harm to an identifiable individual. However, with Biobank there is no special relationship between

---

xviii Human Genetics Commission. Whose hands on your genes? Response document, Liberty, para 6.2.

the participant and the medical researchers. Is a 'special relationship' necessary to establish a duty of care?

In the case of *Tarasoff* v. *Regent's of the University of California* (17 Cal 3d 425 (1976)) a patient told his psychologist that he intended to kill a particular girl. The patient was detained briefly by campus police on the information of the psychologist but was later released and killed the girl. The Supreme Court found that the parents of the girl should have been warned that their daughter was in danger and that liability could not be avoided merely because the victim was not a patient of the therapist.

English courts recognise that for a duty of care to exist there must be a sufficiently proximate relationship[xix] between the claimant (family member who says he should have been warned of genetic risk of serious disease) and the defendant (medical researcher/Biobank). However, 'the more forseeable the harm, the more likely it is that a court will find the relationship between the parties to be proximate'.[15]

Additionally, for a duty of care to exist it must be just and reasonable to impose a duty in the circumstances. In his dissenting judgment in Tarasoff, Justice Clark said that policy issues that determine the duty of care include foreseeability of harm, certainty of the plaintiff's injury, proximity of the defendant's conduct to the plaintiff's injury, prevention of future harm and the burden on the defendant. The Genetic Interest Group stated in 1998 that 'compulsory disclosure of genetic information is unlikely to be justified under the present law'.[13]

The Select Committee (para 280) took evidence that there would be severe difficulties if they had to consult family members – providing warnings to relatives would be time consuming, but it concluded that there are 'very strong moral reasons' for an individual to share information that is potentially life-saving. By consenting to take part in research, particularly non-therapeutic research, it could be argued that there is an altruistic motive on behalf of the research subject that changes the nature of confidentiality.[16]

Personal information may be disclosed without consent, by operation of law – either statute (DPA) or common law (confidentiality). The justification is that there is an outweighing public need for disclosure. Will the Human Rights Act 1998 change the balance given that now the courts are under an obligation to take account of the provisions of Article 8 when interpreting common law?

HUMAN RIGHTS ACT 1998

The Human Rights Act ('HRA') came into force, 2 October 2000. The Act itself states that it gives 'further effect' to the rights and freedoms guaranteed under the European Convention on Human Rights. The UK was an original signatory

---

[xix] In *Palmer* v. *Tees HA* [1999] Lloyds Rep Med 351, Stuart-Smith LJ said 'it is at least necessary for the victim to be identifiable … to establish proximity'.

to the Convention but an individual had to pursue his rights in the European Court. The implementation of the Act means that rights can be secured directly in national courts.

Does the HRA give greater protection to the interests of an individual who has donated his genetic information to Biobank than previously existed under the DPA and the common law duty of confidentiality?

Section 6(1) states that it is unlawful for a *public authority* to act in a way which is incompatible with a Convention right. The Act defines a 'public authority' (s.6(3)) as 'any person whose functions are of a public nature'. In *Poplar Housing and Regeneration Community Association Ltd* v. *Donoghue* [2002] QB 48 it was stated that the definition of what was a public body should be given a generous interpretation. It noted a combination of features that impose a public character or stamp on the body including:

- Funding – 'While the degree of public funding of the activities of an otherwise private body is certainly relevant as to the nature of the functions performed, by itself it is not determinative of whether the functions are public or private' (*R (Heather)* v. *Leonard Cheshire Foundation* [2002] 2 All ER 936 at para 35).
- State function – Is the body standing in the shoes of the state when exercising its function (i.e. the authority) the means by which the state achieves the exercise of its responsibilities towards individuals? Judicial review cases, which are illustrative here, show that a body exercising statutory functions will be a 'public body'. NHS bodies (including NHS genetic testing laboratories – Regional Genetic Centres) are public bodies by virtue of their statutory basis and, for the purposes of the HRA, will be public authorities.

The Lord Chancellor stated that the Act should apply to a 'wide rather than narrow range of public authorities, so as to provide as much protection as possible to those who claim that their rights have been infringed'.[xx] Parliament intended that organisations with a mix of public and private functions (hybrid bodies) would be subject to the HRA in respect of their public functions.

Is Biobank a public authority and therefore required to recognise Convention rights? Although Biobank has no statutory underpinning it does have governmental support and funding (the government is providing £5m – its partners MRC and the Wellcome Foundation are providing £20m each). Given the intention that a wide range of bodies should be subject to the HRA, it seems likely that Biobank will be considered a public authority and will have to act in a way compatible with Convention rights.

However, even a private body may be required to recognise Convention rights. It has always been intended that Convention rights exist to defend the interests of the citizen against the power of the state (personified as public authorities). This is known as the 'vertical effect' of the Act, i.e. the relationship between public authorities and individuals. However, the Act also has a 'horizontal effect' and even private bodies must respect Convention rights.[17]

[xx]In the House of Lords Second Reading of the Human Rights Bill.

This is achieved because courts are public authorities and therefore are required (s.2) to interpret statute and common law in a way that is compatible with Convention rights. This is not limited to situations where the court is reviewing actions of public authorities. There is an obligation on English courts to take account of private and family life under Article 8 when interpreting common law. Therefore if an individual was to challenge the lawfulness of disclosure of his confidential genetic information without consent, the court, in considering the duty of confidentiality, would be required to take account of an individual's right to respect for privacy.[xxi] Convention rights are not directly enforceable against private bodies and to bring Convention rights into play in respect of private bodies there must be an existing cause of action that the court has jurisdiction to hear. If an individual is arguing that his sensitive personal information should not be disclosed under the DPA then the provisions of that Act must be considered in the light of Article 8 and the case law from Strasbourg.

To what extent is it possible for genetic information to be disclosed without consent, contrary to the right to respect for private life?

'The essential object of Art. 8 is to protect the individual against arbitrary interference by public authorities' (*Glaser* v. *UK* [2001] 33 EHRR 1 at para 63).

Article 8 states that everyone has the right to respect for his private and family life. In *Z* v. *Finland* [1997] 25 EHRR 371, it was recognised that protection of personal data is fundamental to respect for family and private life. Article 8 is not an absolute right. A balance is to be struck between 'the demands of the general interest of the community and the requirements of the protection of the individual's fundamental rights' (*Soering* v. *UK* [1989] 11 EHRR 439).

Restrictions on this right to privacy are stated in Article 8(2) – any interference with the right must be 'in accordance with law' and 'necessary in a democratic society' for a 'legitimate aim'.

- In accordance with law – it must be shown that interference with an individual's right of privacy is stated in national law, either statute or common law. As seen above the DPA and the common law duty of confidentiality provide legal bases for interference in particular specified circumstances.
- Necessary in a democratic society – this implies that interference corresponds to a pressing social need and it is proportionate to the legitimate aim pursued. Some relevant legitimate aims (set out in Article 8(2)) include those necessary in the interests of national security, for the prevention of disorder or crime or for the protection of health or morals.

[xxi] In *Douglas and others* v. *Hello!* [2003] EWHC 786 (Ch), Lindsay J declined to hold that there is an existing law of privacy in English law. The law of confidence has expanded to have a similar effect. See *Campbell* v. *MGN Ltd* (Court of Appeal) [2002] All ER 177 at p. 70, for a consideration of the development of 'breach of privacy' and 'breach of confidence'.

A situation might arise where the police ask Biobank to disclose genetic information (DNA sample) to help in the detection of a crime. In considering whether to disclose Biobank would have to balance the individual's respect for private life with the aim of preventing crime.

The case of *Z* v. *Finland* [1997] 25 EHRR 371 concerned a Finnish national whose medical data were disclosed to the police in respect of an investigation of her husband of a series of sexual assaults. The applicant and her husband were both HIV positive. The European Court of Human Rights ('ECtHR') held that the protection of personal data was of fundamental importance to a person's enjoyment of the right to respect for private and family life. Any interference with the confidentiality of such information required to be justified by the overriding requirement of public interest. Here relevant and sufficient reasons showed an overriding requirement of a criminal prosecution.

What about disclosure of genetic information held by Biobank to relevant healthcare authorities, or government/commercial organisations?

In *MS* v. *Sweden* [1999] 28 EHRR 371, an applicant who had injured her back and was unable to work due to back pain many years later made a claim for statutory compensation. In pursuance of the claim it was discovered that the Social Insurance Office had written to the clinic where she had been treated, requesting copies of her medical records and these had been supplied without informing the applicant. Was this a breach of Article 8? The ECtHR held that the disclosure of medical records did amount to an interference with the applicant's right to respect for private life. It did not follow that from the fact she sought treatment at the clinic that she would consent to her records being disclosed for an entirely different purpose of assessing a compensation claim.

However, disclosure was justified under Article 8(2) as being in accordance with the law and in pursuit of the legitimate aim of protecting the economic well-being of the country (disclosure was necessary to calculate the compensation claim). Additionally the Court relied on the fact that the applicant's privacy was respected because the staff of the clinic and Social Insurance Office were obliged by statute to maintain confidentiality.

In *Andersson* v. *Sweden* [1997] 25 EHRR 722, a psychiatrist who considered that a child's health may be at risk because of his mother's health problems, contacted social authorities without the mother's consent. The ECtHR held that disclosure of such data was in conformity with Swedish law, which pursued the legitimate aims of protecting health and morals and the measure was 'necessary in a democratic society'. The restriction on the applicant's right to respect for private life was therefore justified and there was no violation of Article 8.

Proportionate action

Importantly however, the restriction of the right to respect for private life must be proportionate to the aim to be achieved. During the Biobank research, analysis of genetic material may show that a participant has a gene for an inherited medical condition. Is disclosure of genetic information (without consent) to relatives at risk proportionate to the aim of protection of their health?

The case of *Dudgeon* v. *UK* [1981] 4 EHRR 149, illustrates that the more intimate the aspect of private life being interfered with, the more serious must be the reasons for interference before they can be legitimate.

There are three relevant matters to be considered in deciding whether interference with a Convention right is proportionate:

1 whether the objective which is sought to be achieved is sufficiently important to justify limiting the fundamental right. It could be argued that the objective of securing good health is sufficiently important to outweigh an individual's privacy although further advances in genetic research would be needed to show sufficient correlation between the gene and the disease to justify breach of privacy.
2 whether the means chosen are rational and fair and not arbitrary
3 whether the means used impair the right as minimally as possible. Disclosure of risk of genetic disease to the relative's GP, who is under a duty of confidence, would impair the right of privacy in a minimal way (as was recognised in *MS* v. *Sweden*) and may be an appropriate balance between competing interests.

Is there an obligation to disclose to individuals/their relatives that they are 'at risk' of a serious genetic disease under the Human Rights Act?

It is recognised that a state may be liable for violations of Convention rights by private bodies – the state is responsible because it has a duty to prevent the breach (although any remedy would have to be pursued in the European Court not in a national court). This is because there are positive duties on contracting states to secure protection of Convention rights by other individuals (*X and Y* v. *Netherlands* [1985] 8 EHRR 252). Case law shows that there are positive obligations under Articles 2 and 8.

Article 2 states that 'Everyone's right to life shall be protected at law'.

In *Osman* v. *UK* [1998] 29 EHRR 245, Ahmed Osman had been shot dead by his son's school teacher. The question was whether there was a positive obligation to protect his life from the criminal acts of another. The European Court said it was sufficient for an applicant to show that the authorities did not do all that could be reasonably expected of them to avoid a real and immediate risk to life of which they have or ought to have knowledge.

In respect of Article 2, *Osman* provides that the state must take appropriate steps to safeguard the lives of those within its jurisdiction.

However, the positive obligation is not absolute and unqualified. It is necessary to establish two conditions:

1 did the authority know or should it have known of the existence of a real and immediate risk to the life of an identifiable individual *and*
2 did it fail to take reasonable measures that might have been expected to avoid that risk?

Does Article 2 give rise to an obligation on the state to warn of potential health risks? In *LCB* v. *UK* [1998] 27 EHRR 212, the applicant's father had been present on Christmas Island at the time of nuclear testing. The applicant claimed that she should have been warned of her father's exposure to radiation so that she could have sought early diagnosis and treatment of her leukaemia. The issue before the Court was whether the state could reasonably have been expected to provide advice to her parents and to monitor her health – did the state do 'all that could have been required of it to prevent the applicant's life being avoidably put at risk'. The Court concluded unanimously that there was no violation of Article 2. The state would be required to warn the applicant's parents and monitor her health only if it had appeared likely that irradiation of the father engendered a risk to the applicant's health. The causal link between irradiation of the father and the applicant's leukaemia was not established.

In *Guerra* v. *Italy* [1998] 26 EHRR 357, a failure to inform local residents of the hazards of arsenic poisoning from a chemical factory breached an obligation to secure Article 8 rights. The Court found that severe environmental pollution affected individuals' wellbeing and prevented them from enjoying their homes in such a way as to affect adversely their private and family life.

There are difficulties in arguing that there is a positive obligation to warn a participant in Biobank that he has a genetic disorder. First, it would be extremely difficult to show that failure to inform an individual that he has a disease gene would put the individual's life *unavoidably* at risk. For most genetic diseases there is currently no cure and so death could not be avoided even if a warning was given. Second, it could not be said that the risk to life is *immediate.* In The Queen on the application of *DF* v. *Chief Constable of Norfolk Police, Secretary of State for the Home Department* [2002] EWHC 1738, Crane J said that 'immediate' should not be taken to mean that the threat will necessarily materialize in the very near future. Immediacy requires that the risk must be present and continuing (at para 38). Some genetic diseases are of late onset and in many cases, individuals with genetic mutations (such as cystic fibrosis) manifest the disease over a period of time. Third, often the lifestyle/environmental effect on the development of the disease is great and it is not only the provision of information that would prevent the applicant's life being avoidably put at risk – the individual too would have a big part to play in taking steps to ameliorate the disease.

Although with current medical knowledge it may be difficult to show that informing an individual that he has a genetic disease can avoid immediate risk to life, in the future medical research may identify treatments for many genetic diseases and so make the positive obligation to safeguard life a more relevant issue.

Limits to the obligation

In *LCB* v. *UK* it was stated that to establish violation of Article 2 the applicant must demonstrate that advice and information could have altered the fatal nature of her condition or the physical and consequent psychological impact of the disease.

There is no obligation to provide information if it would be futile. 'Futility' is a concept that has been used in the context of the withdrawal of futile treatment. What does 'futility' mean here?

Taken narrowly it would be futile to inform an individual that he has the gene for a late onset untreatable disease because the act of positive obligation would not be life-saving – it would not alter the fatal nature of the condition.

A wider view of the term 'futility' may be that information would alter the physical and psychological impact of a genetic disease if steps can be taken to seek treatment, ameliorate the impact of the disease, or prepare for onset of the disease.

Additionally, the state's positive obligation to safeguard life must be interpreted in a manner that does not impose an impossible or disproportionate burden (*Osman* v. *UK* [1998] 29 EHRR 245, at para 44). Individual participants in Biobank could be identified as the information on the database is not wholly anonymised but it could be argued that to inform relatives at risk may impose a disproportionate burden. The administrative costs necessarily incurred in locating and informing relatives may be prohibitive. There are on average three at risk family members for each patient with a genetic disease[18] and the burden of identifying and tracking down relatives may be too great to justify.

Does a right to respect for private life cover a right not to know?

It is generally considered a 'good thing' to have information about one's genetic inheritance. It enhances autonomy, enabling informed decisions about reproduction, preventative treatment can be sought and appropriate lifestyles adopted. However, this may not be true in all cases. Individuals with severe, late onset diseases, which are untreatable, may prefer not to know. There may be a sense of 'morbidification', waiting for the disease to manifest and potential concerns of genetic discrimination in the workplace and inability to obtain life assurance or health cover. Affected individuals may find reproductive choices onerous.

Genetic testing predicts future events with varying degrees of uncertainty. It would be unduly paternalistic to assume information of a genetic disease should always be disclosed to the individual concerned and of course once the information has been disclosed it is too late to take back.

The right to respect for private life could encompass the right not to receive information about oneself. There would seem to be no justification for breaching that right unless the state could argue that the health of others outweighs an individual's right to privacy, i.e. the right not to be told.

In *Sahin and Others* v. *Germany* [2002] 1 FLR 119, the court said that a parent 'cannot be entitled under Art. 8 of the Convention to have such measures taken as would harm the child's health and development'.

Liberty[xxii] considers that the right not to know should be recognised, qualified in very exceptional circumstances where disclosure to others will protect some other person from very serious harm. Disclosure should be made only pursuant to permission from a judge/judicial body and where disclosure would

---

[xxii] Liberty's Response to the Human Genetics Commission's discussion document *Whose Hands on Your Genes?* at paragraph 6.5, March 2001.

not affect the person concerned, disclosure should be made without overriding the right not to know. By comparison, the HGC[19] prefers the terminology 'an entitlement not to know' recognising that the 'right' not to know may be overridden in certain circumstances.

Article 10(2) of the European Convention on Human Rights and Biomedicine provides that the wishes of individuals not to be informed shall be *observed*. This recognition is not couched in 'rights' language.

CONCLUSION

Whether the protections afforded to genetic information by the Data Protection Act 1998, the duty of confidence and in particular the Human Rights Act 1998 are adequately effective are discussed above. While the latter does offer protection against the disclosure of information without consent, it could be said that the Convention rights are too wide-ranging to adequately respond to the challenge of finely balanced interests posed by the revolution of genetic information.

Individuals taking part in the Biobank study cannot be assured that their genetic information will never be disclosed without their consent. Other interests, including the health interests of relatives may be of sufficient weight to override a participant's right to privacy/confidentiality.[xxiii]

It has been suggested that it is unclear how the defence for disclosure in the public interest would operate.[xxiv]

The notion of 'genetic solidarity and altruism' is proposed by the HGC. This recognises that society is based on mutual cooperation and interdependence and that, from a moral point of view at least, individual fulfilment should not be pursued at the expense of claims of others. Moral claims may not be easily translated into legal principles.

Liberty considers that 'the law could and should go further than it currently does to set the boundaries of unauthorised disclosure of genetic information so that individuals can be aware of what their rights are with some certainty'[xxv] and states that there is an 'urgent need for legislation in this area'.[xxvi]

Some would contend that a genetic privacy law is necessary. Typically such legislation would provide that 'no-one should have or control identifiable DNA samples or genetic information about an individual unless that individual ...

[xxiii] Liberty's Response to the Human Genetics Commission's discussion document *Whose Hands on Your Genes?* at paragraph 2.2. Liberty considers that an individual's right to personal autonomy extends to personal samples and personal information derived from them ... and that there should be 'overwhelming evidence of substantial benefit to society or to other individuals if personal autonomy is to be overridden'.

[xxiv] Liberty's Response to the Human Genetics Commission's discussion document, *Whose Hands on Your Genes?*, at paragraph 6.3, refers to disclosure of genetic information.

[xxv] Human Genetics Commission. *Whose hands on your genes?* Response document, Liberty, para 6.3.

[xxvi] Human Genetics Commission. *Whose hands on your genes?* Response document, Liberty, para 6.4.

has access to and control over the dissemination of that information' (Genetic Privacy Act (US) proposed by Annas, Glantz and Roche, 1995). However, it is usual that there is an exception for researchers to inform 'at risk' relatives.

GeneWatch UK argues that the UK should ratify the European Convention on Human Rights and Biomedicine (ECHRB). The ECHRB deals with non-discrimination on the grounds of genetic inheritance (Article 11) and use of predictive genetic tests (Article 12). Article 10(2) provides that 'Everyone is entitled to know any information collected about his or her health'. Like the HRA however the ECHRB provides for restrictions on rights in the interests of prevention of crime, public health and protection of rights and freedoms of others (Article 26.1).

When asked when the government would sign and ratify the ECHRB the Secretary of State for Health replied that:

> 'The convention covers a wide range of complex ethical and legal issues, many of which have been and remain, actively under debate in the United Kingdom over recent years. The Government wish to consider the conclusions of these debates before reaching a final view on signature and ratification of the convention' (Hansard 20.5.02 col 149W).

Genetic information is becoming more relevant and readily available. Now that genetic testing kits are available directly to the public concerns are raised about voluntary codes of practice and guidance for sale of such tests. It may be increasingly impossible to contain the exchange of genetic information and of greater importance is what is done with the information.

The particular challenge to the expansion of genetic information is that it can be used for controversial purposes such as access to services, insurance and employment. There is a moratorium to November 2006 on the use by insurance companies of predisposition genetic tests for sums insured of over £500 000 for life insurance. However, the House of Commons Select Committee on Science and Technology (5th Report, March 2001) stated that the insurance industry had failed to give clear straightforward information about its policy on the use of genetic test results.

> 'Ultimately the root of the problem does not lie in the accessibility or otherwise of genetic information, but arises because of the discriminatory and prejudicial attitudes within society.'[20]

References

1 Protocol for Biobank UK: A Study of Genes, Environment and Health, The Wellcome Trust, MRC and Department of Health; February 2002.
2 House of Lords Select Committee on Science and Technology, 4th Report – Human Genetic Databases, 20 March 2001.
3 Soren Holm. There is nothing special about genetic information. In: Thompson AK, Chadwick RF, eds. Genetic information: acquisition, access, and control. New York: Kluwer Academic/Plenum Publishing; 1999.

4 Human Genetics Commission. Whose hands on your genes? Response document; Liberty, para 3.3. www.liberty-human-rights.org.uk
5 Human Genetics Commission. Inside information: balancing interests in the use of personal genetic data; May 2002 at 3.33 (Crown Copyright, 27908 1P 6k May 02).
6 Nuffield Council on Bioethics. Genetics and human behaviour – the ethical context. Nuffield: Council on Bioethics; October 2002.
7 Even, arguably, anonymising the information. See Grubb, A. Breach of confidence: anonymised information, case commentary on *R* v. *Department of Health* ex parte *Source Informatics*. Medical Law Review 2000; 8(Spring):115–120.
8 Human Genetics Commission. Inside information: balancing interests in the use of personal genetic data; May 2002 at 3.43 (Crown Copyright, 27908 1P 6k May 02).
9 Kirwan S. Using confidential patient information. Bulletin of Medical Ethics 2002; 174:3–5.
10 Human Genetics Commission. Inside information: balancing interests in the use of personal genetic data; May 2002 at 3.60 (Crown Copyright, 27908 1P 6k May 02).
11 Human Genetics Commission. Whose hands on your genes? Response document, Liberty, para 3.2.
12 Human Genetics Commission. Whose hands on your genes? Response document, Liberty, para 3.52.
13 Genetic Interest Group. Confidentiality and Medical Genetics; 1998:para 2.6.
14 BMA. Human genetics: choice and responsibility. Oxford: Oxford University Press; 1998.
15 Jones M. Medical confidentiality and the public interest. Professional Negligence 1990; 6:16.
16 McHale J. Medical confidentiality and legal privilege. London: Routledge; 1993.
17 Beyleveld D, Pattinson S. Horizontal applicability and horizontal effect. Law Quarterly Review 2002:623.
18 McCrehan Parker C. Camping trips and family trees: must Tennessee physicians warn their patients' relatives of genetic risks? Tennessee Law Review 1998; 65:585.
19 Human Genetics Commission. Inside information: balancing interests in the use of personal genetic data; May 2002 at 3.6 (Crown Copyright, 27908 1P 6k May 02).
20 McGleenan T. Rights to know and not to know: is there a need for a genetic privacy law? In: Chadwick R, Levitt M, Shickle D, eds. The right to know and the right not to know. Aldershot: Avebury.

Chapter 10

Tort law and medical quality: some lessons from the USA[i]

Michelle M. Mello and Troyen A. Brennan

INTRODUCTION

After a decade and a half of quiet slumber, medical malpractice litigation is once again becoming an area of significant interest in health policy. In the USA, this renewed interest arises from the intersection of three phenomena in the healthcare industry: the so-called 'consumer-driven health care' movement and its emphasis on medical quality; the patient safety movement led by

[i]This chapter is adapted from Mello MM, Brennan TA. Deterrence of medical errors: theory and evidence for malpractice reform, © Texas Law Review 2002; 80(7):1595–1637.

regulators, insurers, employers and academics; and a new 'tort crisis' characterised by skyrocketing liability insurance premiums for physicians and hospitals. A key issue in the policy debates over each of these phenomena is the extent to which the tort liability system is effective in deterring medical negligence and improving the quality of medical care.

This chapter examines the available evidence concerning the impact of malpractice litigation on medical quality in the USA. Some limited evidence is found that it deters clinical negligence, but overall, the evidence is thin. The chapter also reviews possible explanations for the weakness of the deterrent signal and suggests a series of tort reforms that could focus deterrence so that it actually does create incentives sturdy enough to improve quality. The conclusion examines the British malpractice system and prospects for improving deterrence in that system along the lines of the suggested reforms.

THE LANDSCAPE OF THE AMERICAN MALPRACTICE ENVIRONMENT AND CONTRASTS TO BRITAIN

The American system for litigating medical malpractice claims differs from the British system for handling claims against National Health Service providers in a number of respects as shown below. It is important to note that there is also a large and growing private medical sector in Britain and the system for litigating claims against those private hospitals and practitioners resembles the American system much more closely.

THE TORT LIABILITY SYSTEM

American medical malpractice law, like British law, revolves around the concept of negligence. A plaintiff in a malpractice case has the burden of proving by a preponderance of the evidence (1) that the relationship between the plaintiff-patient and the defendant-physician gave rise to a duty; (2) that the defendant-physician was negligent – meaning that the care provided fell below the standard expected of a reasonable medical practitioner; (3) that the plaintiff-patient suffered an injury; and (4) that the injury was caused by the defendant-physician's negligence.

Medical malpractice is a matter of state law in the USA and some differences in the standard of care exist across states. Traditionally, the standard of care in a medical malpractice case has closely resembled the British standard in that it has been based on customary medical practice. Now, however, many American states are moving to a more objective 'reasonable prudence' standard. The standard of care in an American informed consent case also varies across states: in most jurisdictions, the scope of a physician's duty to inform patients about material risks associated with proposed treatments is defined by what a reasonable physician would disclose, but a minority of states have moved to a patient-based standard, requiring physicians to disclose all risks that a reasonable patient would expect to be told before undergoing the treatment.[1] The British common-law standard for informed consent mirrors the

American reasonable-physician standard, but the continuing viability of this standard in Britain is unclear in the wake of guidelines issued by the General Medical Council that hew more closely to a patient-based standard.

Several other features of the American tort system diverge from the British system. Each individual defendant in an American malpractice case is responsible for arranging for his or her own defence. Multiple defence attorneys therefore may be involved and may mount separate defences. Each is paid by the physician (through his malpractice insurance premiums) and, in contrast to the British system, legal costs are not reimbursed if the defendant prevails in the case.

Plaintiffs in American malpractice cases hire their own private attorney and nearly all pay their attorneys through contingency fee arrangements, in which the attorney receives a proportion of the damages recovered (up to 40% of the award). In Britain, many plaintiffs qualify for legal representation through the government's Community Legal Service scheme. Contingency fee agreements are considered unethical. However, since 1995 claimants in clinical negligence cases have been permitted to enter into 'conditional fee agreements' (CFAs) in which the attorney takes nothing if the claim is unsuccessful, but recovers his usual fees plus a percentage uplift if the claim is successful. CFAs differ from contingency fees in that the success fee is based on a percentage of the attorney's normal rate, not a percentage of the damages award. Additionally, since 2000, the success fee (if 'reasonable') has been recoverable from the losing party separately from the damages awards, in contrast to contingency fees, which are deducted from the damages award.

The American constitution grants civil litigants the right to a jury trial in matters involving more than a minimal sum of money. Although this right may be waived, most malpractice cases that proceed to trial are heard by a jury. In contrast, British malpractice trials are tried by a judge. In both countries, the overwhelming majority of claims never go to trial. Most are settled, though the likelihood that a plaintiff will receive a non-zero settlement is believed to be higher in the USA than in Britain.

FINANCIAL RESPONSIBILITY FOR MEDICAL NEGLIGENCE

While in Britain the National Health Service (NHS) bears legal and financial responsibility for the negligence of its employees, in the USA, liability for medical negligence is fragmented due to the private and decentralised nature of healthcare delivery. Patients with medical injuries usually sue the individual physicians involved in their care. They may also name a healthcare organisation as a defendant in the lawsuit, but the circumstances in which a hospital or other organisation will be held liable are quite limited. Hospitals are vicariously liable for the acts of their affiliated physicians if they directly employ or control those providers; but most physicians operate as independent contractors rather than employees. Courts have generally limited theories of corporate negligence to cases in which the hospital itself acted negligently, such as in making staff credentialing decisions or setting staffing levels. Thus, although the law in most states provides that physicians and healthcare facilities may be jointly and severally liable for medical malpractice, in practice liability tends to fall heavily on individual physicians.

Except for those who are directly employed by a hospital or health plan, physicians arrange and pay for their own malpractice liability insurance. Hospitals have separate insurance, through commercial carriers, mutual companies formed by several hospitals, or self-insurance arrangements known as 'captives'. Hospital insurance premiums are frequently experience rated to some degree (up to 20–25% above or below the average premium), meaning that the amount hospitals pay is calibrated to their past claims experience. Individual physician premiums vary across clinical specialties according to the risk rating of each specialty. However, physician insurers generally consider it infeasible to individually experience rate their subscribers. Physicians are sued too infrequently and their claims experience varies too much over each 3- or 5-year period, to make experience rating actuarially feasible.

LITIGATION RATES

American physicians are sued much more frequently than their British counterparts. Lois Quam and colleagues have suggested several factors that may account for this disparity.[2] First, British patients who are injured by medical negligence will have their future healthcare costs relating to that injury paid by the NHS, while American patients have no such guarantee. Second, American patients, who pay directly for their health care through monthly insurance premiums or out-of-pocket payments, may be more likely to feel aggrieved when they have a bad outcome. Third, American patients tend to utilise specialist physicians at a higher rate, to have less close relationships with a primary physician and to shift between physicians more often. Therefore, litigation is less likely to disrupt close, longstanding care relationships.

Fourth, plaintiff attorneys are widely available, willing to work on contingency and aggressive in soliciting clients in the USA. In contrast, British plaintiffs have not historically been able to avail themselves of contingency fees or (until recently) conditional fee agreements and not all prospective plaintiffs qualify for Community Legal Services assistance. American plaintiffs who bring unsuccessful cases incur no financial losses, while self-funding British plaintiffs face the prospect of having to pay (through the purchase of insurance) the defence's legal costs if their claim is not successful.

Fifth, the use of juries and the history of generous jury awards in the USA holds out the prospect of enormous recoveries, which serves as a substantial enticement to sue. Sixth, legal rules tend to be more favourable to plaintiffs in the USA. For example, the patient-based informed consent standard is more likely to result in a verdict for the plaintiff than the physician-based standard and American juries are much more willing than British judges to rule for plaintiffs in claims alleging a failure or delay in diagnosis.[3] Finally, Frances Miller has suggested that British patients may be less inclined to sue because they may recognise that damages are paid by the NHS, leaving fewer funds available for medical care.[4] In contrast, the link between malpractice awards and healthcare costs in the USA is less direct, though it is increasingly acknowledged. All of these factors have contributed to high frequency and severity of claims in the USA, periodically leading to periods of 'tort crisis'. Rates of claiming are also rising in Britain, but still do not approach the astronomical frequency and severity of claims of the USA.

With this background in mind, we now turn to a discussion of the functioning of tort law in the USA.

WHAT DO WE KNOW ABOUT THE IMPACT OF TORT LAW ON MEDICAL QUALITY?

According to law-and-economics theory, deterrence is the primary rationale for torts, easily outstripping corrective justice and compensation.[5] The costs of litigation theoretically create an incentive to take safety precautions. This theory rests on some large assumptions, however. With respect to medical malpractice, it assumes that healthcare providers are rational actors who determine their optimal level of precaution-taking on the basis of a careful weighing of the risks, costs and benefits of the various alternatives. Additionally, it assumes that providers actually internalise a significant proportion of the costs of their own negligence – an assumption called into question by the prevalence of liability insurance among physicians and hospitals. What evidence exists that these assumptions hold in American health care and that malpractice litigation does deter medical negligence and improve the quality of care?

MALPRACTICE LIABILITY AND DEFENSIVE MEDICINE

Analyses of the effect of tort liability on medical quality often focus on the phenomenon of defensive medicine. Defensive medicine is care provided primarily to reduce the probability of litigation.[6] Because some of the increase in intensity of health services attributable to defensive medicine is thought to be medically inappropriate, a defensive-medicine response to perceived malpractice risk is really a measure of overdeterrence or excessive precaution-taking, rather than true deterrence of substandard care.

Defensive medicine has long been invoked by chronic defendants (physicians and insurance companies) as a rationale for enacting tort reform. However, the overdeterrence rhetoric has not been firmly grounded in fact. Most defensive-medicine studies have failed to demonstrate any real impacts on medical practice arising from higher malpractice premiums. The now-defunct Office of Technology Assessment of the United States Congress (OTA) comprehensively reviewed existing studies in 1994 and found nothing convincing.[7] In addition to this literature review, it also examined studies of changes in obstetrics access related to malpractice premium charges. Finally, OTA surveyed several thousand physicians using clinical scenarios to elicit their perceptions of defensive medicine. It found some evidence that malpractice concerns spurred defensive practices, but the effect was weaker than previously believed.

Later studies of obstetric care (an area in which defensive medicine is widely believed to be especially significant) have produced mixed findings. Some have found that higher malpractice risk increased the probability of delivery by caesarean section,[8,9] others have found the opposite,[10] and still others have found no association.[11,12] One group of researchers has identified defensive-medicine effects in other clinical settings, but their methods are somewhat peculiar.[13]

It is likely that defensive medicine, to the extent that it ever took place, has diminished over time in response to the growing presence of managed care. In a fee-for-service system, the economic incentive structure encourages defensive medicine, but physicians in capitated practices lose money with each additional service ordered. Even if physicians ignore the economic incentives, their ability to order tests and procedures of questionable medical necessity is increasingly circumscribed by the oversight of cost-conscious managed care payers.

MALPRACTICE EXPERIENCE AND ERROR DETERRENCE

There is little evidence of true error deterrence stemming from medical malpractice liability. Studies of obstetric care have failed to identify any differences in the quality of care rendered by obstetricians with varying histories of malpractice claims. A review of obstetric-care medical records for sentinel markers of errors and other indicators of substandard care found no relationship between the provider having been 'punished' by the malpractice system and having fewer future deviations from the standard of care.[14] Other studies examined the effect of malpractice threat on a range of birth outcomes and found no systematic improvements associated with a physician's prior claims experience.[8,11]

Studies have also been conducted on the relationship between physicians' past malpractice claims experience and their chances of being sued again.[15] It is tempting to view these as deterrence studies as an observed association would seem to suggest that the experience of being punished for negligence reduces the likelihood of further negligence. However, the deterrence question cannot be answered by these studies for two reasons. First, an absence of lawsuits against a physician does not imply an absence of negligence, since only a tiny fraction of patients injured due to negligence file a claim. Second, it might be the case that physicians' perceived malpractice risk exerts a stronger influence on their practice behaviour than their actual claims experience. If so, then studies that focus on the actual claims experience rather than perceived litigation risk as the variable of interest may miss the mark.

Perhaps the most thorough deterrence analysis to date is that performed as part of the Harvard Medical Practice Study (HMPS).[16] The HMPS researchers abstracted information from hospital medical records and malpractice claims files to ascertain rates of hospital adverse events, negligence and malpractice claims in New York in 1984. To examine the deterrence question, the investigators undertook a relatively sophisticated econometric analysis of the association between a hospital's past claims experience and its current patterns of care and adverse events rates. They determined that hospitals facing the highest tort risk had per-patient hospital care costs that were higher than the statewide average, while hospitals with the lowest tort risk had significantly lower per-patient costs, suggesting a deterrent effect.

However, when other measures of the impact of tort risk on medical practice were tried, the result proved unstable. Although the variable representing malpractice risk was negatively associated with the proportion of hospitalisations involving adverse events and the proportion of adverse events involving negligence, the association did not achieve statistical significance at the conventional level. The HMPS investigators struggled with how to interpret these results and ultimately settled on this conclusion: 'Although we did observe the hypothesised relationship in our sample – the more tort claims, the fewer negligent injuries – we cannot exclude the possibility that this relationship was coincidental rather than causal'.[16]

The lack of robustness of the estimates of deterrence is a critical issue. The one HMPS model that did show a pronounced deterrent effect used measures of the intensity of services provided as the dependent variable. Increased *per capita* quantity or cost of services does not necessarily reflect better quality care or lower error rates, however. It may reflect several different phenomena: (1) increased ordering of services that are not medically necessary (defensive medicine); (2) ordering of services that are medically indicated and improve the overall quality of care, but do not effect a reduction in the number of adverse events; (3) ordering of services that do reduce the number of adverse events (deterrence); or (4) ordering of services necessitated by an adverse event. Of these, only the third possibility is an indicator of deterrence.

Recognising the limitations of the initial HMPS analysis, a different subgroup of the investigators later took a second stab at modelling deterrence, incorporating more sophisticated measures of deterrence. They ran a number of different models, which again produced mixed results. A statistically significant negative association (i.e. a deterrent effect) was found for a model using the number of claims against the hospital per 1000 discharges as the malpractice-risk measure and the number of adverse events per 100 hospitalisations as the outcome variable. However, none of the other models evinced a statistically significant deterrent effect. In the end, the investigators were unable to agree on which of the several models was correctly specified or on how to interpret the group of results as a whole. As a result, the findings were not submitted for publication.

The overall picture that emerges from the existing studies of the relationship between malpractice claims experience and medical errors is that evidence of a deterrent effect is (a) limited and (b) vulnerable to methodological criticism. The study findings, while far from solid, are provocative enough to suggest that further empirical study would be appropriate. The findings also raise a question as to why the existing evidence does not provide stronger support for deterrence theory. The remainder of this chapter examines why the deterrent signal may be so weak in American health care and what might be done to strengthen it.

FACTORS CLOUDING THE DETERRENT SIGNAL

Insurance effects

An important factor enervating deterrence is that physicians are nearly universally insured against medical malpractice. The existence of insurance always dampens incentives for taking safety precautions, especially where, as in malpractice insurance, premiums are not experience rated. The possibility of experience-rating individual physicians has been experimented with by a few states and many major insurers, but is generally thought to be unworkable. It is probably impossible to come up with a highly predictive rating formula for individual physicians, because the statistical correlation between instances of negligent care and instances of lawsuits is poor and the degree of autocorrelation in most physicians' claims experience over time is low. Moreover, insurers who have implemented experience rating have found that instead of being chastened by the imposition of higher premiums, physicians tend to simply switch to another carrier if one is available.[17] Thus, the existence of competition among insurers on the open market undermines the possible deterrent effect of experience rating. The situation for hospitals is somewhat different. Because experience rating does occur on a widespread basis for hospitals, the incentive-dampening effect of insurance is a less serious problem than for individual physicians.

The problem of poor fit

Even in a world of perfect experience rating, the deterrent signal would still be blunted by a second problem: the poor fit between instances of negligence and suing. Research has found that most instances of medical negligence never give rise to a malpractice claim and that many malpractice lawsuits are brought and won by patients even though expert reviewers can identify no evidence of negligent care.

The Harvard Medical Practice Study found less than 2% of patients who were injured in the hospital by negligence in New York in 1984 filed a malpractice claim. Additionally, only about one-sixth of all claims filed in connection with hospitalisations in 1984 actually involved both negligence and a cognisable injury.[18] When the HMPS investigators tracked the disposition of the 46 claims closed within a 10-year period, the results were dispiriting: 10 of the 24 cases that expert reviewers judged to have no evidence of an adverse event resulted in a payoff to the plaintiff (mean payment $28 760), as did six of 13 cases judged to involve an adverse event but not negligence (mean payment $98 132). Conversely, four of the nine cases judged to involve negligent injuries resulted in no payoff to the plaintiff. In a multivariate analysis, the presence of negligence was not a statistically significant predictor of the outcome.

Rather, the most important driver of damages was the severity of the plaintiff's injury, whether due to negligence or not.[19]

These findings were validated by a later study of adverse events and malpractice claims in Utah and Colorado.[20] Using 1992 data from 28 hospitals, researchers determined that adverse events occurred in about 3% of all hospitalisations and that about 33% and 27% of adverse events were due to negligence in Utah and Colorado, respectively. Thus, about 1% of hospitalisations involved a negligent injury. When these data were matched against records of malpractice claims filed through 1996 relating to incidents from 1992, it showed that only 2.5% of the patients who were injured due to negligence filed a malpractice claim. In total, the group of patients represented in the sample of medical records reviewed for adverse events filed 18 malpractice claims. The investigators determined that 14 of these claims involved no negligence and 10 involved no adverse event. Only four claims (22%) actually involved a negligent injury. The Utah/Colorado study did not examine payoff amounts and their correlation with negligence.

While there is evidence that those injured due to negligence are more likely than those injured by non-negligent treatment to file a claim, overall these studies do not provide support for the notion that the malpractice system sends a strong deterrent signal to providers. Providers who are negligent face only a small risk of being sued and providers who have not acted negligently cannot feel secure that they will not be sued. To invoke Paul Weiler's analogy of a traffic policeman who allows many motorists who run a red light to pass without giving them a ticket, but gives tickets to many who proceed lawfully through green lights, this mismatch undermines the deterrent signal of the economic sanction.[16]

The problem of externalised costs

Insurance effects and the problem of poor fit combine to undercut deterrence by severely limiting the extent to which the tort system can force hospitals to pay the costs of negligent adverse events. There is no question that medical errors exact a profound societal toll: in addition to their human costs, preventable adverse events in the USA are estimated to produce national economic costs in the range of $17 billion to $29 billion annually.[21] These costs take several forms, including additional acute-care costs, long-term care and maintenance of the disabled, lost income and lost household production. Researchers have attempted to spur cost-minded hospitals to pursue error reduction by disaggregating error costs to the hospital level and arguing that reducing adverse events can save hospitals money. However, such statistics mask the fact that hospitals do not internalise all of these costs.

In fact, most of the costs of errors in the USA accrue to other payers, including private medical insurers, Medicare and Medicaid (the government's health insurance programmes for elderly, disabled and very low-income Americans), state disability and income support programmes and injured patients and their families. There exist only two mechanisms through which hospitals internalise error costs. One is by absorbing the cost of additional medical care necessitated by adverse events. The other is through payments associated with malpractice claims.

It is unlikely that these mechanisms either individually or jointly result in a high degree of cost internalisation. Healthcare costs (including out-patient and long-term care costs) account for only about half of the total cost of errors.[22] Moreover, physicians who are paid on a fee-for-service basis and hospitals that receive *per-diem* payments may be able to obtain reimbursement for many of these care costs from insurance payers. Payments associated with malpractice claims also do not represent a large portion of the cost of errors. Only a tiny fraction of all adverse events due to medical negligence result in malpractice claims and only a fraction of claims filed result in a payoff to the plaintiff. Furthermore, the lack of experience rating in physician malpractice insurance premiums means that providers do not feel the full economic consequences of their mistakes.

In order to improve deterrence, malpractice reforms should be targeted at reducing the extent to which hospitals externalise the costs of medical errors. We now turn to a discussion of particular reforms that would achieve this goal.

SHARPENING THE DETERRENT SIGNAL

An understanding of the theory of tort deterrence and the factors that undermine deterrence provides a foundation for designing a better set of institutional arrangements for improving patient safety. We advocate a shift to a system emphasising greater enterprise liability and characterised by three features: channelling, experience rating and limited no-fault compensation. Channelling refers to the aggregation of individual physicians into larger enterprises – hospitals and hospital networks – by consolidating malpractice insurance coverage in a single carrier. The hospital would cover the cost of malpractice premiums for its affiliated physicians and the insurer would mount a joint defence to claims brought against both the hospital and individual physicians. The hospital's malpractice premium would be experience rated. Finally, a limited no-fault compensation scheme would be implemented, such that claims falling within a predefined class of avoidable adverse events would be automatically paid by the insurer without a formal finding of negligence.

CHANNELLING AND ENTERPRISE LIABILITY

We believe that the key to using malpractice claims as a tool for deterrence is to channel individuals into a larger enterprise, insure hospital and physicians through a single carrier and focus on the organisation or 'enterprise' as the unit of liability. Although relatively few American physicians are direct employees of hospitals, most physicians have an affiliation with a hospital that could be used for channelling. Direct employment or close affiliation with a hospital or larger healthcare system is also becoming increasingly common.

Enterprise liability runs counter to the American tradition of focusing liability on the individual physician, but makes much more sense than individual liability from the standpoint of deterrence. We envision using hospitals or hospital systems as the locus of liability. Others have suggested that managed care plans could serve this role, but with the future of managed care in question, this seems inadvisable. Additionally, hospitals are better situated than health plans to control and change processes of health care, that is, to improve the quality of care and reduce medical errors in response to tort incentives. Because they are chronic defendants, hospitals also are much more likely than individual physicians to respond to the malpractice deterrent signal.

Fully fledged enterprise liability, involving elimination of individual physician liability, is not politically feasible in the USA at this time. However, enterprise liability through channelling programmes is practicable. Existing malpractice arrangements in many American hospitals involve channelling, because there are clear efficiencies in malpractice defence in combining the institutions with the individual physicians. Such arrangements are especially prevalent in university teaching hospitals, where faculties are closely linked to the hospital and healthcare systems. For example, the Harvard Medical Institutions in Boston and the Federation of Jewish Philanthropies in New York already have channelling arrangements in place based on a hospital self-insurance mechanism.[23] There is probably enough channelling in the existing healthcare system to allow certain organisations to undertake a trial of enterprise liability.

EXPERIENCE RATING

Experience rating forms the second key feature of our proposed system. The aggregation of providers into an enterprise is a crucial prerequisite to making experience rating an effective tool for deterrence. As noted earlier, experience rating for individual physicians has been tried and has failed, for very good reasons. Our proposed system would be similar to that employed by leading hospital mutual insurance companies in the USA. Claims against physicians and hospitals would be aggregated on an annual basis. The resulting experience rating for policyholders would be adjusted for hospital-specific risk factors unrelated to provider performance, such as specialty mix, presence of intensive care units and payer and case mix. After this adjustment, it would be possible to identify outliers from the mean and use standard actuarial techniques to calculate premium surcharges or premium returns.

NO-FAULT COMPENSATION

We would advocate a form of no-fault compensation operated by individual insurance companies. We believe it appropriate to compensate and hence deter a subset of iatrogenic injuries both broader and more easily identifiable than the subset deemed to involve negligence. For reasons discussed elsewhere, we would choose the Swedish approach, which compensates those adverse events that are avoidable.[23] Essentially, an injury is compensable under the Swedish system if (1) it resulted from medical treatment, (2) the treatment was medically justified and (3) the outcome was avoidable. These criteria are relatively explicit and are accompanied by over 20 years of precedent directly exportable to the USA.

The difference between a negligent and an avoidable adverse event is critical. The term 'avoidable' is generally used to refer to events caused by one or more errors, while 'negligent' refers to a subset of avoidable adverse events that are the result of substandard care. These definitions do not capture the key distinction, however: the concept of avoidability invokes the idea of error reduction through changes in systems of care, whereas the concept of negligence suggests that errors can be reduced by greater precaution-taking and perseverance by individuals.

Writing 20 years ago, Mark F. Grady recognised, in the legal context, that negligence is not actually a simple matter of personal deficiency or inattentiveness.[24] Rather, as those in the field of engineering have long recognised, all human beings are prone to mistakes. The key is to put systems in place to prevent or mitigate these mistakes. Adopting a systems focus changes our view of the role of negligence. Because the system is designed to prevent or mitigate the effects of instances of individual negligence, the occurrence of an injury due to negligence reflects a systems failure as well as an individual failure.

Using an insurer-based administrative system to identify and compensate the subset of adverse events that are avoidable would reduce the costs associated with the determination of compensable cases, which currently proceeds through a showing of breach of the standard of care in a malpractice suit. Additionally, a focus on avoidable adverse events would overcome the problematic connotations that the concept of negligence has taken on in the minds of healthcare providers. As many writers have made clear over the course of the last 20 years, physicians tend to equate negligence with moral misbehavior.[25] Consequently, they view errors as something to be hidden when they occur.

Other industries in which clients face hazards, such as aviation, have adopted the more constructive approach of considering avoidable adverse events as valuable information to be studied and learned from. Regrettably, in medicine such events are hidden under the cloaks of the peer review and attorney–client privileges. For this reason, a malpractice system that turns on a determination of negligence cannot function effectively as a quality-improvement system that rapidly identifies errors and promotes learning and prevention. Moving to a no-fault system overcomes the problem of moral condemnation and encourages an engineering approach to error prevention.

ANTICIPATING POTENTIAL CRITICISMS

Feasibility of voluntary reform

In the USA, a broad-based move to the type of system we describe is politically infeasible. With the American Trial Lawyers Association a strong lobbying force at both the federal and state levels, it would be impossible to undertake wholesale reform, moving most or all providers to a no-fault/enterprise liability system. However, major insurers, hospitals and health networks could move to an enterprise liability system on a voluntary basis.

We believe many would choose to do so, for two reasons. First, they likely would find that a no-fault/enterprise liability system more readily synchronises with their efforts to improve patient safety. Moving to a system that does not penalise clinicians for reporting adverse events would result in increased reporting and thus increased institutional learning about how to avoid errors in the future. Hospitals will realise cost savings from successful error reduction.

Second, hospitals might find that their customers like the alternative to tort. A health centre could market itself as a responsible institution, committed to providing compensation for avoidable injuries that is prompt, fair and integrated with a physician reporting system. Such an institution would likely be attractive to both physicians and patients. Physicians deeply resent the moral, economic and psychic implications of malpractice litigation and they would respond positively to the opportunity to practice in an environment free of these concerns. Patients likely will also find it attractive to be cared for by hospitals that are committed to speedy reporting of avoidable adverse events, rapid compensation and error prevention programmes.

For these business reasons, we believe there is a reasonable chance that hospitals will wish to participate in a no-fault/enterprise liability system. At the outset, they may have questions, as the liability premiums from the enterprise-based system will be greater than their current premiums. Those using channelling approaches, however, will realise that the premium increase will be addressed by cost shifts between the hospital and its integrated medical staff. Moreover, they should realise that the promise of more patients, along with the increased probability of being able to reduce experience-rated premiums through improved adverse event prevention, more than justify initial costs that may be higher.

Clearly it is unrealistic to expect that all, or even most, hospitals would voluntarily move to our proposed system, especially in the early years when its impacts on costs and market share are unproven. In particular, smaller hospitals that do not find it economically feasible to self-insure for malpractice would be unlikely to move to our system. We also acknowledge that channelling will not work for all physicians. Some solo practitioners who admit patients to several different hospitals will be difficult to tie into a single enterprise.

While these issues are real, it is quite possible that circumstances will change over time. Market trends are tying formerly independent physicians more and more tightly into hospitals and health systems. Market forces also continue to promote consolidation of hospitals and other provider institutions into larger organisations that are more capable of self-insurance and of absorbing a greater proportion of the costs of injuries. Additionally, as evidence regarding the efficacy of an enterprise liability/no-fault system in promoting quality gathers into a critical mass, providers' initial reluctance to move to such a system may be overcome.

Costs of injury compensation

Commentators have identified a series of problems with no-fault compensation schemes for medical injuries, generally focused on the types of payments allowed under existing no-fault systems, the feasibility of such programmes and the method of deterrence.[26] We find these arguments largely unpersuasive. The allowable compensation is a system design feature that can take on many forms and need not reflect existing systems. For example, the system could compensate only for economic injuries related to job loss and medical costs, or it could also compensate for pain and suffering and loss of household production.

We have previously estimated the costs of alternative no-fault schemes for hospitals in New York, Utah and Colorado.[27] This research suggests that it would be possible to compensate many more injuries than are compensable under the current negligence standard and provide a reasonable range of covered losses without increasing the total cost of the liability system relative to the *status quo*. The cost savings arise from a substantial reduction in administrative costs associated with eliminating the negligence determination in malpractice claims. The costs of a no-fault system could be dialled up or down by selecting different definitions of compensable injuries and compensable losses.

IMPACT ON DETERRENCE

Some may argue that moving to an enterprise liability/no-fault system would weaken rather than strengthen deterrence. No-fault is often considered synonymous with no-deterrence, but in fact, most no-fault systems do integrate deterrence through experience-rated insurance premiums. American workers' compensation schemes, for example, have successfully used this mechanism to deter injuries, using the employer as the unit of rating. We believe similar premium structuring could work in medical injury compensation.

By aggregating claims at an institutional level and applying an experience rating, our proposed system addresses the insurance effects that presently obstruct deterrence. Although some experience rating is currently performed for hospitals, the advantage of our system lies in its use of channelling. Rolling the claims experience of a hospital's affiliated physicians into the hospital's own experience rating brings about a clearer picture of the total liability risk associated with care rendered at the hospital. It provides a mechanism for incorporating physician risk information into insurance premiums despite the fact that risk-rating physicians individually is not feasible.

The proposal also addresses the problem of poor fit by introducing an administrative mechanism through which avoidable injuries can be compensated more swiftly and accurately than under the current tort system. By eliminating some of the current barriers to bringing claims, such as the protracted and adversarial nature of litigation, the system increases the likelihood that victims of avoidable adverse events will seek compensation for their injuries.

The system also increases the accuracy of the scheme, i.e. the match rate between cases of avoidable injury and cases in which a payout is made. The problematic notion of negligence is replaced by the more straightforward finding of whether or not the alleged injury fits within predetermined categories of avoidable adverse events. Many of the variables that can lead to inaccurate outcomes at trial, such as the use of hired experts and lay juries, are replaced by a simple administrative system.

The use of an avoidability standard and an administrative claims processing mechanism will result in a greater percentage of avoidable injuries being compensated than are compensated under the present system. Increasing the certainty of the economic sanction for poor-quality care should provide heightened incentives for care improvement. Furthermore, the use of experience rating and channelling makes certain that these sanctions will actually be felt by the providers, rather than simply absorbed by their insurance carriers. Because our proposed system would attack the present barriers to deterrence – insurance effects, the poor fit problem and externalised costs – there is every reason to believe that it would be effective in strengthening deterrence.

One may counter that while a system centred on enterprise liability might increase the deterrent signal for hospitals, it would weaken the effect at the level of the individual physician, resulting in a net loss of deterrence. Several responses to this argument may be made.[28] First, as we have described, there is very little evidence that the current system, with its lack of experience rating, has much of a deterrent effect on individual physicians. It is unlikely that we can do much worse than the status quo. Second, the gains in deterrence at the enterprise-level probably would outweigh the individual-level losses. Hospitals are inherently more attractive targets for deterrence because of their size and resources, their status as chronic defendants and the feasibility of experience rating their insurance premiums. Finally, it is a mistake to view enterprise-level and individual-level deterrence as a zero-sum game. Rather than shielding individual physicians from responsibility for errors, an enterprise liability system will strongly motivate hospitals and health systems to find ways to provide incentives for their affiliated physicians to improve the quality of care.

INCENTIVES TO REPORT ADVERSE EVENTS

We acknowledge that because we incorporate experience rating at the level of the enterprise into our proposed system, the system retains disincentives for individual clinicians to report medical errors and adverse events to centralised reporting systems or hospital peer review and risk management bodies that are in a position to learn from them. Arguably, in our system clinicians will still be reluctant to report errors for fear that their insurance premiums will be hiked up as a result.

We discount this potential impediment for several reasons. First, premiums are rated according to claims experience, not the number of reports made. Only a fraction of reported incidents will end up as malpractice claims.

Second, the individual doctor as reporter will see no change in compensation (or only a very slight change) as a result of any one report to the channelled enterprise. Third, while hospitals will see an increase in premiums associated with an increase in claims, arguably the benefits of knowledge about preventable events outweigh the costs associated with short-term premium increases. This knowledge can be used to design system improvements to prevent error recurrences, which will lead to lower premiums in the long run. Finally, any enabling legislation would have to place additional damages on any no-fault settlement that was not reported by the medical staff (if they should have been aware of it).

IMPLICATIONS FOR BRITAIN

The British National Health Service has avoided many of the pitfalls of the American system of medical justice, but not all. While claim-promoting conditions such as the use of juries and contingency fee arrangements have not been present in Britain, the British system is characterised by many of the deterrence-dampening features we have discussed in connection with American malpractice law. Physicians and hospitals do not internalise the costs of adverse events through experience-rated insurance premiums. Although no HMPS-style data on the match between adverse events and malpractice claiming exist for Britain, it is likely that the problem of poor fit also exists there. There is no particular reason to believe that the care rendered by British providers results in adverse events at a rate markedly lower than that observed in the USA, yet claims rates are far below American rates, suggesting a large pool of uncompensated negligence. In a single-payer system, cost-externalisation does not occur to the extent that it does in the USA, because the NHS absorbs the costs of additional health care necessitated by adverse events. However, individual hospitals and physicians do not internalise these costs.

Finally, Britain, like the USA, relies exclusively on negligence-based tort law to compensate injured patients. British doctors therefore face the same disincentives to report adverse events and errors, with the attendant consequences for learning and systems improvement. The Final Report of the Bristol Royal Infirmary Inquiry recommended that 'In order to remove the disincentive to open reporting and discussion of sentinel events represented by the clinical negligence system, this system should be abolished [and] replaced by an alternative system' of medical injury compensation.[29]

The tort law indeed does not appear to be exerting a powerful deterrent effect on NHS institutions. By March 2000, almost one-quarter of NHS trusts had not attained even the basic risk management standards set by the Clinical Negligence Scheme for Trusts (CNST) and another two-thirds had achieved only the basic standards.[30] Malpractice claims rates in the NHS are on the increase, as are total settlement costs. While these trends may reflect a host of factors other than changes in the incidence of negligence, they are not encouraging.

In view of these problems, the British government recently called for ideas for reforming the handling of clinical negligence in Britain. The Chief Medical

Officer (CMO) released a report in June 2003 analysing the various proposals, including proposals for a no-fault system.[ii] The CMO recommended against adoption of no-fault based on a cost analysis that projected system costs at four to ten times the tort system's current costs. The methodology used to estimate the likely number of compensable claims is, however, somewhat questionable.

While the costs of moving to no-fault in Britain are uncertain, the prospects for implementing such a system are enhanced by the existing administrative structure of the CNST. A stated purpose of the CNST is to create incentives to reduce medical negligence and medical injury. The CNST's voluntary nature, its focus on NHS trusts as the unit of liability and risk management, the National Health Service Litigation Authority's (NHSLA's) power to levy charges on members to cover liability costs and set the amount of those contributions, the CNST's provisions for risk management discounts in those contributions, its claim reporting requirements and the pre-existence of channelling arrangements in the NHS create excellent conditions for a trial of experience rating and no-fault compensation. Claim reporting creates a centralised database of claims information from which experience-rated trust contributions could be calculated. Trusts, which already assume responsibility for risk management and patient safety initiatives, are well situated to respond to the incentives created by experience-rated contributions. The NHSLA is a well-established administrative structure that could centrally receive and process requests for compensation for avoidable adverse events. In summary, the primary barriers to adoption of our proposals in the USA – the decentralised nature of healthcare delivery and liability insurance and political gridlock arising from clashing private-interest lobby groups – do not appear to exist in Britain. The Chief Medical Officer's recommendations notwithstanding, we therefore view the prospects for enhancing the impact of tort liability on medical quality in Britain with considerable optimism.

CONCLUSION

We have proposed liability-based deterrence as a way to build a foundation for quality improvement in health care. If we can reform those aspects of the tort system that presently interfere with the deterrent signal of malpractice litigation and move to a system in which hospitals internalise a greater portion of the costs of errors, we are likely to improve the traditionally troubled relationship between tort law and medical quality. We should focus on evolving the medical liability system beyond negligence-based tort toward an enterprise-based, limited no-fault arrangement in which both physicians and hospitals have incentives for error reduction. For both Britain and the USA, this reform programme, though ambitious, is within reach.

[ii]Chief Medical Officer. Making amends: a consultation paper setting out proposals for reforming the approach to clinical negligence in the NHS. London: Department of Health; 2003.

References

1   Brennan TA. Just doctoring: medical ethics in the liberal state. Berkeley, CA: University of California Press; 1991.

2   Quam L, Fenn P, Dingwall R. Medical malpractice in perspective: II – the implications for Britain. British Medical Journal 1987; 294(6587):1597–1600.

3   Quam L, Dingwall R, Fenn P. Medical malpractice claims in obstetrics and gynaecology: comparisons between the United States and Britain. British Journal of Obstetrics and Gynaecology 1988; 95(5):454–461.

4   Miller FH. Medical malpractice litigation: do the British have a better remedy? American Journal of Law and Medicine 1986; 11(4):433–463.

5   Schwartz GT. Reality in the economic analysis of tort law: does tort law really deter? UCLA Law Review 1994; 42(2):377–444.

6   Office of Technology Assessment. Impact of legal reforms on medical malpractice costs. Washington: US Congress, Office of Technology Assessment; 1993.

7   Office of Technology Assessment. Defensive medicine and medical malpractice. US Congress, Office of Technology Assessment; 1994.

8   Dubay L, Kaestner R, Waidmann T. The impact of malpractice fears on cesarean section rates. Journal of Health Economics 1999; 18(4):491–522.

9   Localio AR, Lawthers AG, Bengtson JM, et al. Relationship between malpractice claims and cesarean delivery. Journal of the American Medical Association 1993; 269(3):366–373.

10 Tussing DA, Wojtowycz MA. The cesarean decision in New York state, 1986: economic and noneconomic aspects. Medical Care 1992; 30(6):529–540.

11 Sloan FA, Whetten-Goldstein K, Githens PB, et al. Effects of the threat of medical malpractice litigation and other factors on birth outcomes. Medical Care 1995; 33(7):700–714.

12 Baldwin L, Hart LG, Lloyd M, et al. Defensive medicine and obstetrics. Journal of the American Medical Association 1995; 274(20):1606–1610.

13 Kessler D, McClellan M. Do doctors practice defensive medicine? Quarterly Journal of Economics 1996; 111(2):353–390.

14 Entman SS, Glass CA, Hickson GB, et al. The relationship between malpractice claims history and subsequent obstetric care. Journal of the American Medical Association 1994; 272(20):1588–1591.

15 Taragin MI, Martin K, Shapiro S, et al. Physician malpractice: does the past predict the future? Journal of General Internal Medicine 1995; 10(10):550–556.

16 Weiler PC, Hiatt H, Newhouse JP, et al. A measure of malpractice: medical injury, malpractice litigation and patient compensation. Cambridge, MA: Harvard University Press; 1993.

17 Sloan FA. Experience rating: does it make sense for medical malpractice insurance? American Economic Review 1990; 80(2):128–133.

18 Localio AR, Lawthers AG, Brennan TA, et al. Relation between malpractice claims and adverse events due to negligence: results of the Harvard Medical Practice Study III. New England Journal of Medicine 1991; 325(4):245–251.

19 Brennan TA, Sox CM, Burstin HR. Relation between negligent adverse events and the outcomes of medical-malpractice litigation. New England Journal of Medicine 1996; 335(26):1963–1967.

20 Thomas EJ, Studdert DM, Burstin HR, et al. Incidence and types of adverse events and negligent care in Utah and Colorado. Medical Care 2000; 38(3):261–271.

21 Kohn LT, Corrigan J, Richardson WC, (eds). Institute of Medicine. To err is human: building a safer health system. Washington: National Academy Press; 2000.

22 Thomas EJ, Studdert DM, Newhouse JP, et al. Costs of medical injuries in Utah and Colorado. Inquiry 1999; 36(3):255–264.

23 Studdert DM, Brennan TA. No-fault compensation for medical injuries: the prospect for error prevention. Journal of the American Medical Association 2001; 286(2):217–223.

24 Grady MF. A new positive economic theory of negligence. Yale Law Journal 1983; 92(5):799–825.

25 Leape LL. Error in medicine. Journal of the American Medical Association 1994; 272(23):1851–1857.

26 Bovbjerg RR, Sloan FA, Rankin PJ. Administrative performance of no-fault compensation for medical injury. Law and Contemporary Problems 1997; 60(2):71–116.

27 Studdert DM, Brennan TA, Thomas EJ. Beyond dead reckoning: measures of medical injury burden, malpractice litigation and alternative compensation models from Utah and Colorado. Indiana Law Review 2000; 33(4):1643–1686.

28 Studdert DM, Brennan TA. Deterrence in a divided world: emerging problems for malpractice law in an era of managed care. Behavioral Science and Law 1997; 15:21–48.

29 The Bristol Royal Infirmary Inquiry. The report of the public inquiry into children's heart surgery at the Bristol Royal Infirmary 1984–1995: learning from Bristol. London: The Stationery Office; 2001.

30 Comptroller and Auditor General. Handling clinical negligence claims in Britain. London: The Stationery Office; 2001.

Chapter 11

Ethics and healthcare resources

Kay Wheat

INTRODUCTION

This chapter examines the ethical issues that arise when demand for health care outstrips available resources. It assumes that healthcare resources are limited and that some form of rationing takes place even if it is not so described. The chapter aims to provide an overview of some of the problems that can arise and some of the ethical viewpoints that can be taken. It might be thought that ethical problems only arise in the context of publicly funded health care, and, indeed, much of the following is concerned with problems thrown up by limited public funding. However, private health care can also raise dilemmas: for example, a private hospital might have several patients waiting for an organ transplant, and although tissue compatibility will probably be the deciding factor in most cases, should there be two or more patients who are a good match with the donor, the decision as to who receives the donor organ will be a non-clinical one. Such a decision will raise ethical problems. There are three ways in which ethical issues can be approached. First, we could examine healthcare provision on a worldwide basis; second, on a national basis, in our case, in the UK; and third, healthcare provision in relation to specific treatments and specific patients. The organ transplant decision falls into the last category.

Worldwide provision of health care relates so much to poverty and the way in which the developed countries' resources might be deployed in developing countries that it is beyond the scope of this chapter to examine this. It will, therefore, concentrate on exploring ethics and the national allocation of resources for health care and on the ethical considerations which arise in connection with specific treatments. One way of describing it is that, in the first area, decisions are made by bureaucrats and, in the second, by doctors. A more sophisticated description is that the first situation is about macro allocation and the second, micro allocation. Macro distribution can also be about how much of a national budget we devote to health care as opposed to education, transport and so on and how we allocate that between regions.

Decisions as to how much should be spent on health care as opposed to other public services are, of course, political decisions and can be made in the light of all sorts of pragmatic considerations. Additionally, the issue of whether to increase public expenditure on any publicly funded service often raises the question of whether this will make any appreciable difference given the way in which the service is administered: for example, the recent reports of the Audit Commission and the Office for National Statistics have questioned whether additional spending is resulting in 'better' health care.[1]

It has been suggested above that worldwide issues are inextricably bound up with issues of poverty, but it would be a mistake to think that poverty is not an issue in the UK. The Black Report raised many links between health and poverty, e.g. reporting that life expectancy at birth was seven years higher in social class one (professional) than in social class five.[2] This is an important factor in deciding how state-provided health care should be distributed. However, it should not be thought that individual treatment decisions do not have wider implications. Take the remarks of an administrator at a London hospital:

'a lady … had a bowel disorder requiring total parenteral nutrition at a cost of £25 000 per annum. She was not from my district so we were cross-charging another district for it, otherwise we would not have allowed her to start treatment. She was in her early thirties, decided she wished to get pregnant so was sent to our IVF unit which made her pregnant with twins. She was admitted for the whole of her pregnancy to ensure the fetuses had optimal growth, went into labour and her twins each spent 6 months in the neonatal intensive care unit before discharge. One died shortly after. We costed the complete episode and it totalled almost £300 000. That meant, in effect, that one of the wards we had closed last year, which would have treated a thousand patients, could have remained open if that had not taken place. I … am certain that many cases like this arise with the various new technologies available.'[3]

The way in which health care is provided (if at all) has always been a concern of medical ethics.[4] However, there are a number of issues that make it of particular concern in the twenty-first century. First, the consumer culture has not developed exclusively in the private sector. In the provision of many public services there is a demand for an acceptable (whatever that may be) level of services. The development of medical litigation in the latter half of the twentieth century has demonstrated that because, ostensibly, it is free, the provision of medical treatment by the National Health Service[i] does not preclude

---

[i] This chapter makes reference mostly to the situation in the UK, but of course many other jurisdictions provide publicly funded health care and the ethical issues raised can be applied to any situation where there is a limitation, financial or otherwise, on healthcare provision.

'consumer' demand, both in terms of quality and availability. Second, life expectancy is increasing, and there is concern about the demands on health care by the elderly.[3] Third, technological advances mean that there are treatments available, often expensive treatments such as organ transplants, in situations where previously there were none.

There are three key ethical issues discussed in this chapter. One issue is whether there is a fundamental entitlement to a basic level of health care, regardless of the ability to pay. There might be pragmatic disputes as to what constitutes a 'basic level' of care, but that does not alter the general ethical argument, although it might, in another context, be interesting to compare differing views from the standpoints of economics, sociology, and culture. This raises another key issue, which concerns whether, once this basic threshold has been passed, we can ethically justify the grounds upon which non-basic treatments should be provided. In other words, there is an assumption that healthcare provision is finite and is never sufficient to match the 'needs' of patients. This assumption might be challenged on the basis that health care is so fundamental that society should make available the resources necessary for all patient needs and that creating this dichotomy between basic and non-basic needs is begging the question, and the wrong question at that. This is a rational ethical position to take, but it ignores the fact that resource allocation is an issue in practice and that ethical dilemmas result from this. Furthermore, it side-steps discussion of the other of the three key issues, i.e. the important question of what constitutes a healthcare 'need' in the first place.

WHO NEEDS HEALTH CARE?

The answer, of course, is that only the sick need health care, i.e. only those who are ill, or lack 'health'. The World Health Organization has described 'health' as 'a state of complete physical, mental and social well-being and not merely the absence of disease or infirmity'.[3] A tall order indeed: what proportion of the world could be described as being 'healthy' in the light of this definition? On the flipside of the coin, various attempts have been made to define 'illness', 'disease' and so on.[5] These relate to the manifestations of the condition, i.e. distress, discomfort, etc., but these reactions can be made to many conditions for which there is no underlying pathology. To simply say, however, that there must be an underlying pathology or whatever, is unhelpfully saying that they are caused by illness or disease. Another approach is to say that there is some form of deviation from the 'norm', but that can raise serious issues as to how the 'norm' is defined. This can be particularly problematic in cases of mental illness. Feeling 'unwell' is often no help in psychiatry, as, for example, some schizophrenic patients feel extremely well at a time when they are most likely to harm themselves. In psychiatry the boundary between health and sickness can become very blurred indeed. Ian Kennedy gives the example of the American Psychiatric Association deciding by a vote whether homosexuality was a 'psychiatric condition', i.e. an illness.[6] The provision of treatment for infertility is another difficult issue, as infertility is not generally regarded as an illness, despite the fact that it would undoubtedly qualify as 'ill health' under the World Health Organization's definition. Furthermore, the developments in genetics, which open up the possibilities of using genetic manipulation to eliminate certain physical characteristics such as baldness, surely cannot be said to be dealing with a condition of, or causative of, ill health. Such developments might give rise to objections that they are really about eugenics and that 'improving the human race' is condemnatory of the diversity of people.[ii] Defining a healthcare need is not only problematic in these dramatic examples. The same sort of problem can arise in the case of very mundane forms of treatment, for example, surgery to correct minor physical defects such as the removal of benign and painless cysts. Further, if one favours a definition of ill-health that categorises it as a degree of deviance from the 'norm', it is easy to see how people who might be genuinely untroubled by a condition would nevertheless not wish to be described as 'abnormal'.

A RIGHT TO BASIC HEALTH CARE?

The concern here is not with rights in the sense that they might be protected by, for example, the European Convention on Human Rights, but about the ethical arguments, which could support such a right, rather than presupposing that such a right exists. Leaving aside for the moment the question of how we define basic health care, we can probably assume that it would cover 'nursing care', i.e. the provision of necessary hydration, nutrition and warmth. Many might argue that it would also cover pain relief, although clearly there are many pain-relieving drugs and procedures, and the decision as to what form pain relief might take can slip over into a decision about resource allocation. It is also arguable, however, that life-saving treatments should also come under this heading. One of the justifications for maintaining a right to a basic level of treatment might be that it is akin to having an ethical obligation to rescue when there is no or little risk to oneself.[iii] However, the right to basic nursing care cannot be justified under this heading as it would apply to someone very close to death who could not be 'rescued'. The better view is that it is about respect for human dignity in the sense proffered by Kant: human beings should never be regarded as merely a means to the ends of others, but must be regarded as ends in themselves and therefore deserving of respect.[7] On this basis it could be argued that human beings have a right to an irreducible minimum of nursing care and pain relief. There are many different forms of pain relief, so perhaps it should include at least generic analgesics and minor surgery. However, this might be too simplistic. In a western society where medical treatments and care are much more sophisticated, there is a strong argument for insisting that the 'basic' level should include much more. In turn, however, this means that 'basic' rights are different

---

[ii] See, for example, The Times, 24/4/03, where Nobel prize winner Professor James Watson stated that this sort of 'political correctness' was stifling genetic advancement.
[iii] There is no legal obligation under English law to rescue, even if there is no risk to oneself, unlike some other jurisdictions, for example, French law.

depending upon whether the patient is in the UK or Ethiopia, and this does not sit easily with the language of rights, which tends towards universalisation.

Similarly, the rescue argument applies to care that might be much more sophisticated and costly than nursing care, and this ethical obligation is, again, based on the value of human beings *per se*. At what point is the obligation to rescue no longer applicable to someone in need of, say, expensive life-saving surgery? The problem can be shelved for the time being, however, as arguably, either the 'rescue' will be a short term holding operation, which can be regarded as basic health care, or it will take the form of a treatment which has to be allocated to some, but not all patients.

NON-BASIC HEALTH CARE – WHO GETS IT?

We are not here concerned with only life-saving treatment. On the contrary, a lot of potentially life-saving treatment might come into our first, basic, category, e.g. a right to a well-equipped and widely available emergency ambulance service, a right of reasonable access to healthcare facilities with good resuscitation equipment and so on; in other words, the 'holding operation' facilities previously referred to. At first glance it might be thought that we made a mistake with our categorisations here, and that all life-saving procedures should be in the first category and only non-life saving procedures should be in the second. Sometimes reference is made to essential and elective medical procedures; again, the argument might be made that our first category is about essential, and the second is about elective, procedures. The task of healthcare allocation would be easier if the categories could be defined in these ways. However, such an approach ignores too many of the ethical dilemmas. The patient of 98 who will die without a heart transplant operation would then fall into our first category, i.e. the patient who is claiming a right to basic health care (leaving aside the question of the availability of a suitable heart). Conversely, a patient of 50 who is immobile and in crippling pain due to an arthritic hip would be in the non-life saving, or elective category. It might be possible to sustain an ethically sound argument in support of the 98-year-old's surgery, but is it helpful to base that argument upon the essential/elective dichotomy? Similarly, non-life saving health care might well fall into the first category inasmuch as it could be argued that a sick patient whose survival is not threatened should, nevertheless, be entitled to basic nursing care as part of their right to respect for their human dignity.

At some point in a discussion of medical ethics the tension between a consequentialist approach such as utilitarianism and individual rights emerges and allocation of healthcare resources is no exception. However, as Dickenson argues, if maximisation of welfare is the test, i.e. a basic utilitarian analysis, then a lot of vulnerable people will miss out on medical treatment.[8] On the other hand, a rabidly individualist approach is graphically illustrated by the following recent example. It concerns a 9-year-old child who suffered from a rare form of haemophilia which does not respond to Factor VIII, the blood clotting agent used by most haemophiliacs. In consequence, his doctors adopted a course of treatment to try to make his body respond favourably to Factor VIII. The treatment lasted for 11 months and failed. The cost was £2 million. A heart bypass operation costs £5000, a hip replacement operation costs £4000; both operations have very high success rates, yet there are waiting lists for these procedures. Richard Nicholson, editor of the Bulletin of Medical Ethics, said 'There is a very real problem with the way our society tends to make the individual paramount because this gives comfort ... to doctors who wish to spend whatever it takes to try and heal individuals'.[9]

Dickenson[8] examines the sort of criteria that can be used to allocate resources. First, clinical criteria; second social criteria and finally criteria which are based upon some form of 'equality'. She subdivides the clinical criteria into those based on diagnosis and those based on prognosis. The diagnosis test is that the patient is allocated resources based upon medical need, whereas the prognostic approach is based upon the best chance of recovery. It is interesting to question how the concept of triage fits into this. This concept was developed in the context of military action where the wounded would have to be assessed very quickly. They would fall into one of three categories: those for whom treatment would be futile; those who would survive (at least in the short term) without any treatment, and those who would only survive if treatment were given immediately. Those in the last category are the only ones to receive treatment on the battlefield. Although this is an idea that has been usefully adopted in accident and emergency departments, it has its limitations in non-emergency situations. Some clinicians might like the idea of arranging their waiting lists this way (it might work for example in cases of non-emergency life-threatening conditions, e.g. those needing heart bypass surgery, who may need it with varying degrees of urgency). However the Journal of Medical Ethics[10] reports an interesting experiment which casts doubt upon this form of assessment. Drs Parsons and Lock surveyed British nephrologists by describing 40 of their own patients (anonymously of course) and asking them to select 30 of them for dialysis. The description would include their sex, marital status, age, home facilities, underlying disease, and additional disease. The task therefore was to reject 10 of the patients. It was shown that of the most commonly rejected patients, at least six of them had been successfully treated by Parsons and Lock in their own unit and not one of the patients was rejected by everyone. One of the nephrologists could not find any valid reason to reject any of them.

Dickenson cites the case of a patient at the Churchill Hospital in Oxford, who she describes as a 'vagrant'. He was on dialysis, but this was terminated on the basis that he was not capable of following a diet and other requirements for successful treatment.[8] Clearly, from the strict medical perspective, he was as suitable for dialysis as any other patient so that his rejection was on the basis of his 'personality'. No doubt it would have been described in terms of whether he would benefit from the treatment (an old chestnut used with good effect in many medical law cases, e.g. *Airedale NHS Trust* v. *Bland* [1993] AC 789), but it must be said that if he was lacking in terms of his mental capabilities, he should have been treated in his best interests anyway (see for example *Re F (Mental Patient: Sterilisation)* [1990] 2 AC 1). It must then be the case that, on this test, he should have received the dialysis treatment.

Dickenson's social criteria are based either on past merit – 'social worth' – or future merit, which would be about their potential contribution to society. To use such criteria at all is surely offensive. Certainly, these sorts of considerations rule out a lot of disabled or poorly educated people. It is a double tragedy for the people concerned: they are disabled, poor, unemployed, mentally ill and so on, and because of this they are going to be denied medical treatment. Harris cites the moral distastefulness of this sort of 'double whammy' in relation to denying people treatment on the basis that they are terminally ill: 'Because I have once been unlucky I am no longer worth saving'.[11] He uses this to suggest that greater weight might be given to the shorter life. Harris also pursues a number of anti-ageist arguments in this vein, arguing that whatever our age, we have the rest of our lives to live.[11]

The third category, that of distributing health resources on the basis of 'equality' raises some interesting questions. General notions of equality are fairly meaningless: it is hard to escape the viewpoint that you only treat people equally when you treat them according to their need, and then we find ourselves looking once more at how we prioritise need. Nagel, in a discussion of the concept of 'equality' cites the example of two siblings. One is healthy and happy, the other suffers from a painful handicap. Their parent is about to change jobs and has the choice of moving to an expensive city where the disabled child would receive special medical treatment and schooling but where the family would live in an unpleasant environment, or to a semi-rural location where the other child would be able to pursue his hobbies of sport and natural history. If they move to the country, the healthy child will receive a benefit only if things are made worse for the disabled child. Nagel argues that an improvement in the situation of the disabled child is more important than the same improvement or even a greater improvement for the healthy child.[12]

However, a more robust approach can be taken: we can treat patients like participants in a game of chance and draw lots to decide who to treat. This has been done in practice. Beauchamp and Childress cite the examples of the distribution of drugs to treat multiple sclerosis and AIDS; once patients had achieved the threshold of very basic medical criteria the drugs were distributed by lottery.[13] Another way of doing this is by use of waiting lists, i.e. first come, first served. This is impartial and non-judgemental.

Some might argue that in order to make ethical decisions in the area, one should be looking at what accords most with justice. It could be said that this is about treating patients with equal respect, but, again, this does not help us in deciding whom to treat. John Rawls is probably the most well known exponent of a liberal theory of justice, what he calls 'justice as fairness' and he is famous for his 'veil of ignorance' test.[14] He was trying to reconcile two, ostensibly incompatible positions. The first is that people are basically self-interested and, second, that it is desirable nevertheless to adopt a system of distributive justice. The scenario he asks us to imagine is this: we are aware of the way our western economic system works, but we are in ignorance of the place we occupy in the hierarchy of wealth. In this state of ignorance we have to formulate a system of distribution of the economic benefits and burdens. Although we are basically selfish, Rawls's view is that we would devise a system to ensure that those people at the bottom of the pile have a decent life because we might turn out to be one of those people. Clearly, his view is based upon another assumption: we are not serious gamblers, and are naturally risk-averse persons.

A fierce debate took place between John Harris and John McKie and others[15–19] about a Rawlsian approach to resources and, in particular, in relation to the 'quality adjusted life year' (QALY). An invention of the economists, the application of QALYs makes a valiant attempt to provide a mechanism, albeit an unsophisticated one, for deciding how to ration scarce health resources. Newdick describes it as follows:

> 'It asks (i) to what extent, and for how long, will a treatment improve the quality of a patient's life and (ii) how much does the treatment cost. In this way it seeks to compare the costs of generating QALYs, regardless of the particular treatment in question. In this theory, there is a sliding scale on which each year of full health counts as one, and each year of declining health counts as less than one; death scores 0 … The theory favours treatments which achieve the greatest increase in the quality of life, over the longest period, for the least cost.'[3]

Little more than a superficial glance tells us that there are lots of definitional problems to grapple with here. What is full health? What is declining health? This is just as problematic if comparisons are being made between patients who are seeking the same treatment, or radically different treatment. Newdick cites the example of a patient who is confined to a wheelchair, and who is effectively competing for treatment with a so-called able-bodied patient. The first patient will always score lower than the second. Apart from the legal issues that might arise in relation to disability discrimination, ethically there can be no justification for this as it means that the first patient's life is inherently less valuable than that of the second. McKie argued that patients behind a Rawlsian 'veil of ignorance' would choose QALYs to determine how medical treatment was allocated, because QALYs maximise utility, so 'self-interest' is here being defined in the wider sense. Harris argued that by applying Rawls's argument to QALYs, the result would be that, given the choice, a person would prefer a shorter, healthier life to a longer one in severe discomfort and disability, but he is not convinced by this. Furthermore, he maintains that a person's life would be valued more even if the difference in life expectation is very small, so that in deciding who gets the valuable treatment, someone who would survive for just a few days more than another would get the treatment. Harris argues that all needy people would get the treatment, and McKie points out that this would mean that someone with a 30-year survival expectancy would be treated the same, i.e. not receive priority treatment, over someone who would only survive for a few days. The debate was largely unresolved, but both Harris and McKie object to any form of allocation that would create social divisiveness.

Another factor is the issue of who takes the decision. Doctors will tend to fight their corner. Their specialties are their babies (almost literally in the context of IVF treatment which has a glamorous and competitive side to it), and they will want to further their field of medicine. Would committees made up of laypersons make a better job of resource allocation? The Oregon experiment is one of the best known of a number of surveys of public opinion in this area. A Health Service Commission was established to rank various treatments in order of priority, partly on the basis of public opinion, canvassed by means of questionnaires, but also at public meetings which, despite being open to all, were usually attended by those employed in the healthcare system.[3] Perhaps most people would rather leave these things to 'the professionals', and perhaps there is a serious risk of prejudice (another survey found that people would only consider treating AIDS patients if they were 'innocent' victims[20]) although the termination of dialysis treatment for the 'vagrant' clearly indicates that prejudices are not confined to non-clinicians.

References

1 Hawkes N, Duncan G, Bennett R. Hospital targets under fire as extra cash goes to waste. The Times, 5 June 2003.

2 Black D, Towened P, Davidson N. Inequalities in health: The Black Report. Harmondsworth: Penguin; 1990.

3 Grant K. The balance of care provision in the National Health Service. In: L'Etang H, ed. Health care provision under financial constraint: a decade of change. Royal Society of Medicine; 1990:138, quoted in Newdick C. Who should we treat? Oxford: Clarendon Press; 1995:7, 8, 21, 22, 30.

4 Mason JK, McCall Smith RA. Law and medical ethics. London: Butterworths; 1991:4.

5 Culver CM, Gert B. Philosophy in medicine. New York: Oxford University Press; 1982:66.

6 Kennedy I. The unmasking of medicine. London: Allen & Unwin; 1981:1.

7 Paton HJ. The moral law. London: Hutchinson University Library; 1948.

8 Dickenson D. Is efficiency ethical? Resource issues in health care. In: Almond B, ed. Introducing applied ethics. Oxford: Blackwell; 1995.

9 Dobson R, Rogers L. Boy has £2 m of drugs on NHS. The Sunday Times, 20 April 2003.

10 Gillon R. Editorial. Journal of Medical Ethics 1980; 6:171.

11 Harris J. The value of life. London: Routledge; 1985:89.

12 Nagel T. Mortal questions. Cambridge: Cambridge University Press; 1979:123.

13 Beauchamp TL, Childress JF. Principles of biomedical ethics, 5th edn. Oxford: Oxford University Press; 2001:268.

14 Rawls J. A theory of justice. Oxford: Oxford University Press; 1972.

15 Singer P, McKie J, Kuhse H, Richardson J. Double jeopardy and the use of QALYs in health care allocation. Journal of Medical Ethics 1995; 21:144–150.

16 Harris J. Double jeopardy and the veil of ignorance – a reply. Journal of Medical Ethics 1995; 21:151–157.

17 McKie J, Kuhse H, Richardson J, Singer P. Double jeopardy, the equal value of lives and the veil of ignorance: a rejoinder to Harris. Journal of Medical Ethics 1996; 22:204–208.

18 Harris J. Would Aristotle have played Russian roulette? Journal of Medical Ethics 1996; 22:209–215.

19 McKie J. Another peep behind the veil. Journal of Medical Ethics 1996; 22:216–221.

20 Tomlin Z. Their treatment in your hands. The Guardian, 29 April 1992.

Chapter **12**

Regulating the quality of health care through Judicial Review

Duncan Pratt

CHAPTER CONTENTS

INTRODUCTION

The story of Judicial Review of health care is largely the story of challenges to the allocation of resources, whether that relates to refusals of treatment, or to closing or altering the character or units, or to inadequacies of infrastructure. Where there are funding constraints, priorities of spending must be established. The High Court has a limited but developing role to review how the National Health Service and other healthcare providers perform that function.

The High Court's reviewing jurisdiction has further been engaged in recent years to determine questions arising out of ethical considerations (such as the management of issues about the creation and termination of human life, and embryo research) and liberty of the subject (Mental Health Act powers). The scope of those discrete issues demands a work more extensive than this chapter to do them full justice.

Judicial decisions affecting the allocation of resources carry their own risks. Intervention in one meritorious cause may produce unfairness and unlooked-for consequences elsewhere. Courts have expressed unwillingness to substitute their own judgment for those of the proper authority on the basis that they are not equipped to do so. But courts can and do understand the *process* by which decisions are made and are much readier to interfere where the process or reasoning was defective. The role of the law to interfere has grown but remains limited. It is primarily aimed at securing consistency, transparency and the avoidance of capricious decisions.

The judicial toolkit employed includes the normal principles of statutory interpretation, requirements of rationality and *Wednesbury* reasonableness and (with some caution) legitimate expectation. The toolkit is of course now expanded to include the overarching requirements of the articles of the European Convention on Human Rights (ECHR) introduced by the Human Rights Act 1998.

THE BROAD NHS FRAMEWORK

Some elements of the statutory framework, within which Judicial Review of decisions may be made, are worth identifying. Some are direct but most relevant powers are delegated. The effect of delegating his powers is that the Secretary of State has, for the time being, divested himself of those powers, save to the extent that he has expressly reserved any powers for himself: *Blackpool Corporation* v. *Locker* [1948] 1 KB 349 at 377–378. The Secretary of State has statutory power to give directions to health authorities, special health authorities, primary care trusts and NHS trusts (see s.17 NHS Act 1977, as substituted by Section 12 of the Health Act 1999) and those bodies in turn have a duty to comply with them (see s.126(3)(c) of the NHS Act 1977). In reality, directions are rarely given. Guidance is frequently given. It represents a more attractive option for a Health Secretary who may want to distance himself from the political responsibility for decisions, and is likely to be more flexible in practice. The disadvantage is that compliance cannot be directly compelled. However, government may employ indirect steps to bring a defaulter into line, for example in allocation of budgets. Just as importantly, the existence of guidance may give the patient a basis for seeking Judicial Review on the ground of a fundamental failure of the decision-making process, the thwarting of a legitimate expectation, or that it is *Wednesbury* unreasonable (sometimes also put in other ways, such as unintentional perversity, or implicit error of law in failing to take the guidance properly into account). Such an example is *R* v. *N. Derbyshire HA* ex p. *Fisher* [1997] 8 Med LR 327 – the Beta interferon case. Dyson J held that a health authority's policy for deploying that drug in the treatment of patients suffering multiple sclerosis was unlawful because it failed to give serious consideration to the advice offered in the relevant NHS circular. The circular required them to develop and manage the entry of such drugs into hospitals. The judge was satisfied that the health authority's policy in fact amounted to a blanket ban on the use of the drug, in this particular case. The persistent battle between the cost and efficacy of such drugs has not gone away.

The national healthcare system is a creature created by statute and statutory instrument, and that framework reflects financial constraints and priorities. One theme of Judicial Review decisions is that the duty to provide and the right to receive healthcare benefits is not to be regarded as absolute, even where there is apparently unconditional statutory language. This is most vividly illustrated by the court's interpretation of the statutory cornerstone of the whole system in Section 1 of the National Health Service Act 1977, which sets out the duties of the Secretary of State:

'to continue the promotion ... of a comprehensive health service'.

'When exercising his judgment he has to bear in mind the comprehensive service which he is under a duty to promote as set out in section 1. However, as long as he pays due regard to that duty, the fact that the service will not be comprehensive does not mean that he is necessarily contravening either section 1 or section 3 ... a comprehensive health service may never, for human, financial and other resource reasons, be achievable ... '

'In exercising his judgment the Secretary of State is entitled to take into account the resources available to him and the demands on those resources.'

(In *R. v. North and East Devon Health Authority*, ex p. *Coughlan* [2000] 2 WLR 622; [1999] Lloyds Rep Med 306, Lord Woolf MR construed the statutory duty at 314.)

The courts have traditionally regarded judgments made by the Health Secretary, in purported execution of this duty, as a political question for which judges are not equipped. There is a now an identifiable degree of willingness to scrutinise his reasons and the coherence of those reasons, but assuming proper advice, the Health Secretary should readily jump through that hoop.

Health authorities (or the various successor trusts which arise, disappear and multiply with bewildering rapidity) exercise specified health functions on behalf of the Secretary of State, but at the heart of the statutory scheme, budgetary constraints are now to be found, and reinforce the instinctive approach of the Courts:

'It is the duty of every [Health Authority and Primary Care Trust] in respect of each financial year, to perform its functions so as to secure that the expenditure of the trust ... does not exceed [its income]': Section 97A and D of NHS Act 1977.

Since April 2002, we have had about 330 health authorities in England and Wales in place of the 100 larger authorities, and the government proposes a further reorganisation, which may create yet further, and powerfully independent authorities. Against this background it is likely that existing distinctions in practice and priorities between one area and another will increase. The role of guidance (designed to achieve consistency where appropriate) and the way the Courts approach that guidance, are likely to become more important. Most recently a high profile source of guidance emanates from the National Institute for Clinical Excellence (NICE). It is an instrument for achieving consistency, but it is specifically subjected to budgetary considerations by an amendment to its governing instrument, introduced soon after its creation:

'Subject to and in accordance with such directions as the Secretary of State may give, the Institute shall perform such functions in connection with the promotion of clinical excellence *and of the effective use of available resources* in the health service as the Secretary of State may direct':

(Reg. 3 of National Institute for Clinical Excellence (Establishment and Constitution) Order SI 1999 No. 220 as amended by SI 1999 No. 2219.)

CHALLENGING DECISIONS IN THE COURTS

Treatment

In regulating the quality of health care, decisions about giving or withholding treatment by health authorities, rather than by individual doctors, are likely to have more important consequences for the operation of the system. Nevertheless, to the individual patient it does not matter who took the impugned decision. The principled reluctance to interfere with decisions about spending priorities is very evident in judgements about decisions by health authorities about making treatment available, but important developments have nevertheless occurred, both in the common law and in applying the ECHR.

Common law

In dealing with such decisions by individual doctors, two important principles are established at common law. First, a doctor cannot be compelled to give treatment which he is unwilling to give because it is against his clinical judgement: *Re J (A minor) (Child in care: medical treatment)* [1993] Fam 15. Second, a doctor is not under a duty to provide or continue treatment which has become futile, or is not in the best interests of the patient, even where such treatment would prolong life and death will result from its withdrawal: *Airedale NHS Trust* v. *Bland* [1993] AC 789; *NHS Trust A* v. *Mrs. A and others* [2001] Lloyds Rep Med 28. The last-mentioned case also considered important ECHR arguments to which I shall return. Are there any limits to the protection offered by these principles? If the question has been referred to the court and awaits a full hearing, it would be wrong to withdraw treatment pending that decision. Does a doctor who holds a minority view, particularly if based on ethical rather than clinical grounds, have a duty to make his patient aware of the availability of doctors with an opposite point of view? Such an argument has failed in a negligence claim (see *Burr* v. *Matthews* [1999] 52 BMLR 217) but may be open to argument. Taking this into the wider context, it may be that a health authority whose resources include doctors who would be willing to give the treatment might be obliged to facilitate a referral to such a doctor.

But if the patient is competent, no question of 'best interests' can arise, and the patient is at liberty to refuse the treatment. This was demonstrated in a vivid context in *St. George's Healthcare NHS Trust* v. *S* [1998] 2 FLR 728, where a pregnant mother who had rejected medical advice to have an urgent caesarean delivery because she had developed pre-eclampsia, so putting at risk not only her own life but also that of her baby, was held to have been unlawfully admitted and detained under the Mental Health Act and unlawfully forced to have a caesarean section by order of a judge at first instance. Pregnancy did not diminish a woman's entitlement to decide whether to undergo the treatment and an unborn child's need for medical assistance did not prevail over the mother's rights.

Treatment may be withdrawn because it has achieved its intended purpose, or because it is no longer beneficial, or because authority for the treatment is withdrawn. It is obvious that the first two may involve clinical judgement, to which normal *Bolam* principles will apply.

Before the introduction of the Human Rights Act, the common law had developed principles for reviewing decisions by health authorities to give or withhold treatment. A case which is much revisited in subsequent decisions, and therefore influential, is *R v. Cambridge DHA*, ex p. *B* [1995] 1 WLR 898 – a leukaemia case. Sir Thomas Bingham MR, overturning the judge's original decision to quash a health authority's refusal to fund a third course of chemotherapy and a second bone marrow transplant, said:

> 'difficult and agonising judgments have to be made as to how a limited budget is best allocated to the maximum advantage of the maximum number of patients. That is not a judgment the Court can make. In my judgment, it is not something that a health authority … can be fairly criticised for not advancing before the Court.'

It is to be noted that the original judge (Laws J) acknowledged that the court should not make orders with consequences for the use of health service funds in ignorance of the knock-on effect on other patients but justified it in this case because '*[the Health Authority] must explain the priorities that have led it to decline to fund the treatment*' and found it had not adequately done so here. That approach is more consistent with the way the court *now* reviews decisions. Whatever the individual merits of the outcome of ex p. *B*, it would be a rash health authority who declined treatment without producing reasons which demonstrate it has considered the material factors.

That modern approach can be seen in the more recent decision of the Court of Appeal in *North West Lancashire Health Authority v. A, D and G* [2000] 1 WLR 977; [1999] Lloyds Rep Med 399 – the transsexuals case. The decisions of the health authority to refuse gender re-assignment treatment were quashed, because:

1 Although the health authority was entitled, in establishing its own funding priorities from finite sources, to give greater priority to life-threatening and other grave illnesses than to others less demanding of medical intervention, it must:
   a accurately assess the nature and seriousness of each type of illness
   b determine the effectiveness of various forms of treatment for it
   c give proper effect to that assessment and determination in the formulation and individual application of its policy.

2 The health authority's policy was flawed in this case because:
   a it did not treat transsexuality as an illness, but as an attitude of mind that did not warrant medical treatment
   b the ostensible provision made for exceptions in individual cases and its manner of considering them amounted effectively to the operation of a 'blanket policy' against funding treatment for the condition because it did not believe in such treatment.
3 The stance of the health authority, coupled with the uniformity of its reasons for rejecting each of the patient's requests for funding was not a genuine application of a policy subject to individually determined exceptions.

Arguments were also advanced on behalf of these patients under the ECHR, Articles: 8 (right to private and family life), 3 (right not to be subjected to inhuman or degrading treatment) and 14 (right not to be subjected to discrimination). They were dismissed as adding nothing to the consideration of adequate and more precise domestic principles, and the successful patients were deprived of one-third of the costs they would normally be awarded to reflect the time taken up arguing these unhelpful points. This was hardly a welcoming embrace from our domestic courts for Human Rights Act principles in this area.

However, with or without the assistance of Convention rights, the willingness of the courts to require the basis of a decision to be opened up to scrutiny makes it likely that some older cases would not be decided in the same way today. For example, R v. *Central Birmingham Health Authority*, ex p. *Collier* [1988] unreported save in Kennedy & Grubb[1] but which attracted much press interest at the time, concerned a child who was at the top of a list for life-saving heart surgery. His operation was postponed on several occasions. The court accepted that the defendant had sound operational reasons to bump the child off the operation list, without subjecting that decision to the degree of scrutiny which would now be required following the transsexuals case.

A patient who seeks higher priority for treatment than another will still encounter formidable difficulties, even in the mental health context, as is illustrated by R v. *Oxfordshire Mental Healthcare NHS Trust and another*, ex p. *F* [2001] EWHC Admin 535. In that case, a patient sought to overturn a decision by the defendant's 'Priorities Forum' (a panel including clinical experts) refusing particular treatment which had been recommended by her responsible medical officer (RMO) allocated to her because she was compulsorily detained under the Mental Health Act. Her lawyers argued (among other things) that because of the RMO's role and responsibility under the statutory scheme, his clinical judgement should be determinative of the question unless it were irrational, or at least should be followed in the absence of a compelling case to the contrary. The Forum's decision was a funding decision, balancing the interests of this patient against those of other patients including those who had psychiatric treatment needs but were voluntary patients. Sullivan J held that the health authority owed the same 'target' duty under Section 3 of the National Health Service Act 1977 to those who suffered physical or mental illness and the fact that this patient was under compulsory detention did not alter that underlying target duty. The Mental Health Act 1983 did not expressly provide an enhanced duty towards those compulsorily detained, and no such duty could be implied. The RMO's position under the 1983 Act did not propel his detained patients to the head of the treatment queue. It was for the health authority to decide what weight to give his view. It had reviewed and given weight to it, albeit concluding that there was no clinical consensus as to the correct treatment. The judge observed:

'I acknowledge that the *Wednesbury* threshold is a very difficult one for claimants to overcome in the field of resource allocation, but that is precisely because of the highly judgmental character of such decisions, involving as they do the weighing of numerous, often conflicting, interests, where there will be no single "correct" answer.'

Applying convention rights

Depending on the context, Articles: 2 (right to life), 3 (prohibition of torture or degrading treatment), 5 (right to liberty and security), 8 (respect for private and family life), 12 (right to marry and found a family) or 14 (prohibition of discrimination, so long as the facts also fall within one of the other articles) may be engaged. This chapter is concerned with Judicial Review in the domestic English courts, but a short and necessarily incomplete excursion into decisions by the European Court of Human Rights may indicate some of the ways in which those articles have been applied and which are now available to be urged on the domestic courts.

Article 2 confers a right to life and imposes an obligation on the state to take appropriate steps to preserve life. But it is not to be interpreted as imposing an impossible or disproportionate burden on the authorities. Accordingly not every claimed risk to life gives rise to a Convention requirement to take measures to prevent that risk from materialising: *Osman* v. *UK* [1999] 1 FLR 193 para 116. Article 2 was earlier considered in *Association X* v. *UK* [1978] 78 DR 78, a claim brought by parents whose children had suffered severe permanent injury or death as a result of a voluntary vaccine programme in pursuance of a policy to eliminate or substantially reduce a serious illness in the population. It was found that the case was inadmissible on the facts because the state had taken 'appropriate steps' with a view to the safe administration of the scheme, which was sufficient to comply with its obligation to protect life. It is a necessary inference that, but for such a system of administration, there would have been a breach of Article 2. The European Commission (now absorbed into the Court) has been prepared to assume that Article 2 could be interpreted as imposing on states the obligation to cover the costs of medical treatments including medicines essential to save life (*Scialacqua* v. *Italy* [1998] 26 EHRR CD 164) but it is difficult to foresee the circumstances in which even this generous view may give rise to successful claims by individuals. If an express right to treatment were read into Article 2 (or 3), the courts are very likely to follow the interpretation of a similar constitutional provision by the South African

Constitutional Court, which refused to interfere with the prioritisation of spending on different forms of treatment in a claim brought by a patient needing kidney dialysis: see *Subramoney* v. *Minister of Health* (*KwaZulu-Natal*) [1997] 4 BHRC 308, 313–314, para 19. In *LCB* v. *UK* [1999] 27 EHRR 212 the daughter of a RAF serviceman who had been on Christmas Island during nuclear testing, complained of a breach of Article 2 by failing to take appropriate measures to protect her life, by advising her parents to monitor her health on account of a risk transmitted from her father. The duty to give such advice would only have arisen if it appeared likely (at that time) that her father's exposure to radiation 'might have engendered a real risk to her health'. On the facts, the state ought not then to have been aware of that risk. But again, the inference is that if the state was or ought to have been aware of the risk, there was a duty, derived from Article 2, to provide medical advice and care to the individual.

Article 2 is not at odds with the common law principles outlined above. It does not prohibit the withdrawal of life-prolonging treatment where such treatment ceases to be in the best interests of the patient: *NHS Trust A* v. *Mrs M and others* [supra]. The court decided that so long as the responsible clinical decision to withhold treatment is in accordance with a respectable body of medical opinion, the state's obligation under Article 2 is discharged. It does not impose an absolute obligation where such treatment would be futile. Furthermore, Butler-Sloss P, giving the judgment of the court, drew a distinction between a deliberate act and an omission (see para 30 of her decision). In her view, the phrase 'deprivation of life' must import a deliberate act, by someone acting on behalf of the state, which results in death. A responsible decision by a medical team, based on clinical judgement, not to provide treatment, is not caught. The patient's death is then the result of the illness or injury. In the President's view, the situation was the same where there was a decision to discontinue treatment which is no longer in the best interests of the patient and would therefore be a violation of his autonomy, even though that discontinuance will have the effect of shortening his life. 'Autonomy' is a term increasingly deployed when analysing patient rights in the context of healthcare treatment (see below). She went on to hold that an omission to provide treatment by the medical team will only be incompatible with Article 2 where the circumstances are such as to impose a positive obligation on the state to prolong the patient's life. Presumably the English courts would therefore have no difficulty with the unreported decision of the Commission in *Widmer* v. *Switzerland* [App 202527/92] that Article 2 does not require that the state should make 'passive euthanasia' (by withholding treatment) a crime.

The Court of Appeal went a step further in *Re A* (*conjoined twins: separation*) [2001] 2 WLR 480. It held that the intention to take a life, against which the state is obliged by Article 2 to provide protection, applies only to cases where the purpose of the prohibited action is to cause death, and not to acts or omissions which have as their purpose the saving of a life, but where another death may be an unwished-for consequence (see, for example, Robert Walker LJ at 589H–590A). A necessity had arisen, to avoid inevitable and irreparable evil. That involved choosing between the conflicting duties to the two conjoined children. Article 2 did not in these circumstances import any prohibition, additional to that under the English common law, to the proposed operation. So long as the purpose of the action was not to cause death (notwithstanding that the death of one twin may be an anticipated if unwanted consequence) criminal intent was not present. Going on to consider that the proposed operation was a positive act of invasive surgery, Ward and Brooke LJJ held that the court had to strike a balance between the interests of each twin and do what was best for each by considering the worthwhileness of the proposed treatment, and the advantages and disadvantages of giving or withholding it. That balance came down in favour of the one twin whose body was capable of obtaining advantage from the treatment.

Deriving principle which is of useful application to other cases from the anguished decision in the *conjoined twins* case is a difficult matter, and it may not be useful to attempt to do so. But speculation necessarily arises as to whether the defence of 'necessity' to what would otherwise be medical murder has given rise to new considerations in clinical decisions. Suppose a clinician has an existing elderly patient on a heart lung machine, but that patient has a short life expectancy and poor prospects for his quality of life. A young patient arrives, who would derive more benefit in terms of life expectancy and quality of life, if treated with the same machine. Does any decision whether to switch the machine now permit consideration of the competing interests of the two patients? Formerly, the only interests to be considered were those of the elderly patient. Probably, the answer is that the quality of inevitable and unavoidable necessity is absent.

The meaning assigned to 'degrading treatment' under Article 3 by the ECHR in *Ireland* v. *UK* [1978] 2 EHRR 25, is 'ill treatment designed to arouse in victims feelings of fear, anguish and inferiority, capable of humiliating and debasing them and possibly breaking their physical or moral resistance'.

In regulating healthcare provision, the *withholding or withdrawal* of treatment may amount to a breach of Article 3. So in the healthcare context, the Commission found a breach of Article 3 in *Hurtado* v. *Switzerland* [1994] A/280-A (unreported) where a criminal suspect, with a fractured rib, was not X-rayed or treated for 6 days. In *D* v. *UK* [1997] 24 EHRR 423 a breach of Article 3 arose from a threat to deport a patient who was receiving life-prolonging treatment for AIDS in this country, to a country in the West Indies where such treatment was not available and would therefore hasten his death. The decision was said to arise from the exceptional circumstances of the impact on D's fatal illness, and so far as I am aware no commentator has concluded that it foreshadows an absolute right to continued medical treatment. If withdrawal will lead to death, it may engage, but there is nothing in the ruling that limits engagement of Article 3 to cases involving the threat of death (as opposed to some other serious irrevocable consequence).

Interesting issues have arisen in the application of Article 3 to cases involving patients under a disability, often mentally ill patients. A recent case in which the Court of Appeal expressly applied a decision of the European Court of Human Rights is *The Queen, (N)* v. *Dr M and others* [2003] Lloyds Rep Med 81.

The domestic court adopted the standard of proof required to show medical necessity as set out in *Herczegfalvy* v. *Austria* [1992] EHRR 437:

> 'as a general rule, a method which is a therapeutic necessity cannot be regarded as inhuman or degrading. The court must nevertheless satisfy itself that the medical necessity has been *convincingly shown* to exist.' [emphasis added]

The court said the answer to that question will depend on a number of factors, including (a) how certain it is that the patient does suffer from a treatable mental disorder; (b) how serious a disorder it is; (c) how serious a risk is presented to others; (d) how likely it is that, if the patient does suffer from such a disorder, the proposed treatment will alleviate the condition; (e) how much alleviation there is likely to be; (f) how likely it is that the treatment will have adverse consequences for the patient; and (g) how severe they may be. The court then went on to apply its earlier decision in *Re S (Sterilisation: Patient's Best Interests)* [2000] 2 FLR 389, holding that whether the treatment satisfies the *Bolam* test is a necessary, but not a sufficient condition of whether treatment is in a patient's best interests. Determining best interests may involve choosing the best option between a number of options, all of which satisfy the *Bolam* test (see paras 28 and 29 of the judgment). In this case, however, the patient had obtained an independent clinical opinion to the effect that she did not require the proposed treatment, to which she did not consent. The court rejected the submission that where there is a responsible body of opinion that a patient is not suffering from a treatable condition, then it *cannot* be convincingly shown that the treatment proposed was medically necessary, describing that proposition as 'in effect, a reverse *Bolam* test'.

In mental health, the clinical and judicial elements of health care are closely interwoven because of the elements of restraint and forcible treatment. Article 5 of the Convention has been recently applied by the English courts to review judicially the practice of Mental Health Review Tribunals in delaying listing of applications for the review of compulsory detention or repeatedly adjourning them: see *R (C)* v. *London South West Region Mental Health Review Tribunal* [2002] 1 WLR 176 (CA) and a decision by Burnton J (*R* v. *Mental Health Review Tribunal and another,* ex p. *KB and others* [2002] EWHC 639 (Admin)), where the court's willingness to intervene contrasts markedly with its unwillingness to intervene in healthcare priorities and spending. Burnton J held that although normally questions of financial policy fell within the Executive's remit and not the court's, when issues were raised under Articles 5 or 6 of the Convention, the court could be required to assess the adequacy of resources and the effectiveness of administration. The correct approach was to consider whether the requirement of a speedy hearing had been breached and then for the Health Secretary to discharge the onus of proving that the delay was excusable. It is difficult to see why the court is equipped to adjudicate on this allocation of resources and not on others.

The same judge was called upon to determine the lawfulness of a seclusion policy in managing a patient detained under the Mental Health Act: *S* v. *Airedale*

NHS Trust [2002] EWHC 1780 (Admin). He held that no infringement of Article 3 would arise from its short term use, and even where it was not used as a short term or emergency measure, there was still not necessarily an infringement, because it would not necessarily reach the required level of seriousness. Nor did a breach of Article 5 arise from proof of unnecessary seclusion, since it affected the terms of a person's detention, but did not amount to detention as such. The intellectual flexibility involved in these conclusions may be better understood against the actual facts that seclusion was used for this violent patient who was prone to abscond, because no bed was available at a secure hospital, and the alternative was to enable him to go out into the community.

Article 8 (the right to respect for private and family life) is not often at the heart of decisions by the courts on challenges to healthcare decisions about *physical* illness. But in another case arising from the Christmas Island radiation exposure, the applicants relied on a breach of Article 8, in failing to give them access to health information so as to enable them to assess the possible consequences of exposure for their own health. The court found Article 8 applicable and that a positive obligation arose under it, where a state engaged in hazardous activities which might have hidden adverse consequences on the health of those involved, to provide effective and accessible procedure to such persons to seek relevant and appropriate information. On the facts, however, that duty was adequately discharged: see *McGinley and Egan* v. *UK* [1998] 27 EHRR 1.

More frequently, Article 8 is engaged when considering decisions about *psychiatric* illness. Bizarre facts may therefore arise. In *R* v. *Ashworth Hospital Authority*, ex p. *E* [2001] EWCA the question was whether the Article 8 rights of a male patient, detained in a special hospital, were infringed by refusing to allow him to dress as a woman. At common law, it was held that implied statutory powers had been exercised for the purpose of detention and treatment in accordance with *Wednesbury* principles, but that there had been an admitted infringement of his rights under Article 8(1) of the Convention. That was justifiable and therefore lawful because the restrictions reflected a pressing social need and were proportionate to the legitimate aims pursued. The underlying message is again that health authorities must be able (whether or not through clenched teeth) to demonstrate a reasoned and intelligible basis for the management or treatment decision.

FACILITIES AND ORGANISATIONAL PROVISION

It is in the context of challenges to decisions about healthcare facilities that the case of *Coughlan* (supra) may be placed, but the same approach of principle is to be found as in consideration of treatment decisions. *Coughlan* concerned the closure of a purpose-built home, managed by the local NHS trust, in which the appellant, a tetraplegic requiring regular catheterisation and suffering breathing and mobility problems, was accommodated. A promise of a home for life had been given to the appellant, which raised a legitimate expectation of a continuing substantive benefit. In considering the propriety of the decision to close the home notwithstanding the promise, the court looked to see if the health authority had identified other needs and factors, which outweighed the promise. It held that the health authority had failed to weigh the conflicting interests correctly and there was no overriding public interest which justified frustrating the appellant's legitimate expectation. Therefore the decision to move her was unfair and an abuse of power, in the absence of an offer of accommodation which was reasonably equivalent.

A recently reported case extends these principles, which evolved in the context of NHS health care, to patients detained at *private* psychiatric hospitals: *R v. Partnerships in Care Ltd* ex p. *A* [2002] 1 WLR 2610. The claimant had a severe personality disorder. She required treatment including psychotherapy in a therapeutic setting. She was detained in a private psychiatric hospital run by the defendant, where a unit with such facilities existed. Her treatment was funded by the health authority. She sought Judicial Review of the decision to alter the focus of the unit away from dealing with patients with a personality disorder, so that in future it would serve women with a primary diagnosis of mental illness. Treatment would consist mostly of medication. Preliminary issues were heard as to whether the hospital managers were amenable to Judicial Review and whether the defendant was a 'public authority' within the meaning of Section 6 of the Human Rights Act 1998, and therefore prohibited from acting incompatibly with the claimant's Convention rights. Keith J ruled that such a decision was an act of a public nature (there was a public interest in the hospital's care of persons detained there), that the hospital managers were a public authority within the meaning of the Civil Procedure Rules and Human Rights Act, and that their decision was amenable to Judicial Review. It is tempting to consider this as a case where the new HRA law, and the definitions imported by that Act have informed the approach to domestic Judicial Review jurisprudence.

Nor is it sufficient for a health authority to go through the motions of a bogus consultation exercise in order to arm itself against challenge to a decision for the removal of a facility: in *R v. North and East Devon Health Authority* ex p. *Pow and Ors* [1998] 39 BMLR 77, Moses J decided that the authority was under a duty to leave sufficient time for consulting the public and the local Community Health Council prior to making decisions.

Nevertheless, so long as the appropriate decision making process is adhered to, and it withstands scrutiny on the grounds mentioned above, a health authority is entitled to take into account a lack of funds. In the analogous field of local authority services, the House of Lords has confronted the question: What, if any, limitations can be placed on a duty to assess a disabled person's needs (s.2(1) of the Chronically Sick and Disabled Persons Act 1970)? In *R v. Gloucestershire County Council* ex p. *B* [1997] AC 584, it was argued with apparent logic that a person's needs depended on the nature and extent of his disability; on which question the local authority's resources were irrelevant. Lord Nicholls said at 604E:

'This is an alluring argument but I am unable to accept it. It is flawed by a failure to recognise that needs for services cannot sensibly be assessed without having some regard to the cost of providing them. A person's needs for a particular type or level of service cannot be decided in a vacuum from which all other considerations are expelled.'

Cases about the withdrawal of facilities are fact-sensitive, and the scope of the duty should not be too widely expressed; see *R* v. *Brent, Kensington and Chelsea and Westminster Mental Health NHS Trust* ex p. *C* [2002] LTL 18/2/2002. It was found that, on the evidence, the trust did not promise the applicants a home for life at a particular mental health unit, which was never intended to be other than an interim facility. Tellingly, there was a finding that the trust had considered their needs honestly and reasonably throughout in an attempt to provide suitable accommodation and care. So the court appears to have considered material which satisfied the requirements in the transsexuals case. The judge also held that the trust was required to act compatibly with Article 8, but the applicants' Article 8 rights were inextricably bound up with the trust's primary obligation to provide medical care, and the proposed changes were desirable for their benefit. A failed challenge to proposals to reconfigure the provision of health services in East Kent (*R* v. *E Kent Hospital NHS Trust and another* ex p. *MS* [2002] EWHC 2640 (Admin)) nevertheless demonstrates that the court received and carefully evaluated evidence of the consultation process and the changes to a plan which had been made in consequence. The courts are now entirely comfortable with this reviewing jurisdiction, but it does not follow that the results go all one way.

Whether a treatment or drug is made available at all is a matter in which government has a keen interest, because of the cost implications, but may wish not to take political responsibility for denying access to what is often seen by the public as a modern drug miracle. Statutory bodies have been established to advise the Health Secretary, and he in turn has usually deployed the tool of issuing guidance, rather than directions (see above). The courts have been called upon to review such guidance and its effect: *R* v. *Sec of State* ex p. *P* [1999] Lloyds Rep Med 289. This concerned a Department of Health circular containing guidance from the Health Secretary's advisory committee to GPs not to prescribe Viagra routinely. It is necessary to bear in mind that GPs enjoy great clinical freedom to prescribe drugs they consider necessary for their patients' treatment:

> 'a doctor shall order any drugs or appliances which are needed for the treatment of any patient to whom he is providing treatment': NHS (General Medical Services) Regs 1992, SI 1992 No. 635, schedule 2, para 43).

This is subject only to statutory controls of formally embargoed drugs ('the black list') and those which are restricted ('the grey list'). In the Viagra case, the departmental circular was held to be unlawful, because it was an attempt to circumvent the normal lawful statutory process (i.e. the statutory use of the 'black list' by the Minister) and its effect, expressed in mandatory terms, was to place GPs in breach of their terms of service (by restricting the exercise of their duty under para 43). Collins J held: 'Paragraph 43 … is dealing with the mechanism to enable a patient to receive a drug if the doctor decides that that drug should be used to treat the patient ... The doctor *must give such treatment as he, exercising the professional judgement to be expected from an average GP, considers necessary and appropriate'* [emphasis added] per Collins J at 295. And further '... the evidence confirms that this [circular] was and is intended to be acted upon by GPs independently of whether in their professional judgement a patient needed ... Viagra. Thus I am satisfied that the circular was and is unlawful' (p. 296). The Secretary of State then exercised statutory powers to place Viagra on the grey list. However, that was not the end of the story because the drug company challenged the lawfulness of restricting the drug in that fashion. The Health Secretary justified doing so because of competing priorities for NHS resources. The challenge was on the basis that his decision did not contain a statement of reasons based on objective and verifiable criteria and was this in breach of EC Council Directive 89/105/EEC on the transparency of measures regulating the pricing of medicines. Turner J and then the Court of Appeal dismissed the challenge, holding that the Directive did not require the Health Secretary to conduct an in-depth analysis, and a requirement for transparency was satisfied (*R v. Sec of State for Health* ex p. *P Ltd.* [2002] EWCA Civ 1566).

No doubt the limits of the detail of reasoning, which must be shown, will continue to be worked out. The first instance judge in the Viagra case applied the observations of Sir Thomas Bingham in ex p. *B* (supra), so we see how the European and domestic strands of judicial thinking have gone on to feed, support and occasionally modify each other. The judicial toolkit is considerably expanded by the introduction of Convention rights, but they are more readily adopted when they can be accommodated within the stream of common law thinking.

Reference

1   Kennedy I, Grubb A. Medical law, 3rd edn. London: Butterworths; 2000:340.

Index

Note: Page numbers in **bold** refer to boxes, figures or other non-textual information.

D

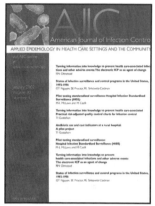